The Right Start

The Right Start

Guidelines for Your Baby's Nutrition and Lifelong Health

by
MARCIA E. YOUNG
and
MICHAEL W. YOUNG

Walker and Company
New York

First published in the United States of America in 1987 by the Walker Publishing Company, Inc.

Published simultaneously in Canada by Thomas Allen & Son Canada, Limited, Markham, Ontario.

Library of Congress Cataloging-in-Publication Data

Young, Marcia E., 1942–
The right start.

Includes index.
1. Infants—Nutrition. 2. Infants—Health and hygiene.
I. Young, Michael W., 1951–   . II. Title.
RJ216.Y68   1987   613.2'024042   87-16068
ISBN 0-8027-0968-0
ISBN 0-8027-7305-2 (pbk.)

Printed in the United States of America

10 9 8 7 6 5 4 3 2 1

Book design by Manuela Paul

To our children, Becky and Mike,
who were the inspiration for this book

TABLE OF CONTENTS

TABLE OF CONTENTS

Caution

This book is based upon our professional experiences and studies of the scientific literature. It is not intended, nor should it be regarded as, medical advice. It is a guide to nutritional disease prevention for healthy people. Please consult with your physician before making any major changes in your eating habits.

FOREWORD

Parents have been feeding children successfully through the ages without the benefit of books like this. Intuition, common sense, and Mother Nature—except in the face of real deprivation—seem to prevail. When help is needed, then the wisdom of the ages, advice from relatives and neighbors, and books and articles on infant care are available. Unfortunately, the available advice in today's world is often inadequate, inappropriate, or even wrong.

Medical research has made great strides in the last twenty years and the fund of knowledge about pediatric nutrition continues to expand. There are numerous application of this knowledge that can promote healthy growth and development. There is, as well, considerable evidence that certain disease processes, such as atherosclerosis, can be prevented, or halted, by nutritional modification in the child's early years.

Pediatricians and other health-care professionals are becoming increasingly concerned about the prevalence of chronic disease in children. Some chronic pediatric problems, such as obesity, are complex, and have organic and social determinants, but are nevertheless often approachable through appropriate feeding practices. Other problems such as food sensitivities that can arise from interactions between diet and physiological processes, can be alleviated by careful attention to what the growing child eats.

THE RIGHT START is a comprehensive and responsible effort to integrate new information about pediatric nutrition into everyday family practice. The authors have taken care to present widely accepted, and some not-so-widely accepted, theories and to make recommendations in a straightforward manner. Their practical advice in the form of tips and recipes add to the immediate usefulness of the book.

They make no claim that sorting out today's welter of information and misinformation about children's diet will be easy. Nevertheless parents and others will find an abundance of help here. It is becoming increasingly apparent that what we don't know or fail to apply about basic nutrition may in fact hurt our children. What we learn and apply into their daily lives can be of lifelong benefit to them.

George A. Little, M.D.
Professor, Dartmouth Medical School
Chairman, Department of Maternal & Child Health
Dartmouth-Hitchcok Medical Center
Hanover, New Hampshire

INTRODUCTION

If you've selected *The Right Start* from all the other baby feeding books available to you, chances are you're a smart, forward-looking parent. There are many books that will teach you the basics of infant nutrition or baby food making, but *The Right Start* is the first book to include comprehensive infant-feeding guidelines incorporating the latest findings in nutritional research and disease prevention. It is the only book that helps you apply the exciting recent discoveries in nutritional disease prevention to your infant and your whole family so that you may all enjoy many healthy, happy years together.

Much has been learned about the foods we eat and how they effect our health. Nutritional factors have now been identified that increase our risk of developing cancer, heart disease, atherosclerosis, hypertension, allergy, and obesity. Other factors have been identified that can actually protect us from these diseases. By learning which foods to avoid and which foods to add to our diets, we can optimize our health and actively defend ourselves against disease. The nutritional information that we present represents a synthesis of the latest findings of such well-respected organizations as the National Academy of Sciences, the National Institutes of Health, the American Academy of Pediatrics, the American Heart Association, the American Cancer Society, and others. Within the last few years, these major medical and scientific institutions have uncovered definitive links between many diseases and the foods we eat. Some of this information may seem revolutionary because of its remarkable promises of health and longevity, but all is well grounded in scientific fact and has been published by the more conservative of scientific organizations.

Researchers in the fields of medicine and nutrition are now enthusiastically looking forward to an era of preventive measures that will profoundly enhance the quality of life and longevity of anyone who is willing to participate. As individuals, we need only apply these simple new dietary guidelines to our own lives to begin to reap the benefits of better health and even reverse the course of many disease states. As parents, we have the opportunity and the responsibility to extend these promises of health and longevity to our children, who stand to gain the most from such a program. Their bodies have not yet been compromised by years of poor eating habits, and their minds are not yet set into patterns which may have to be changed.

But there are other important reasons to begin disease prevention with our infants. Most parents are unaware of the far-reaching health effects of infant feeding. For example, allergic disease, which is the cause of chronic suffering for 20 percent of the population, has its roots in early infant feeding. Allergists will tell you that formula feeding and early introduction of solid foods are the prime initiators of allergies. Feeding your baby the wrong foods, at a time in his* life when he's not mature enough to handle the challenge, can provoke a life-long allergic condition in him, even if your family has no history of allergy. *The Right*

*For simplicity of language, we have used the male pronoun throughout this book. Perhaps this is because our new son dominated our lives during the writing of this book.

Start provides you with detailed guidelines for food introduction that will avoid triggering allergic reactions and minimize your baby's risk of ever developing an allergy.

It may seem odd to be discussing diseases such as heart disease, atherosclerosis, hypertension, and obesity in a baby feeding book. After all, they are diseases that generally become apparent in middle to later life. However, physicians are now coming to realize that these disease states begin their destructive processes early in life. A recent government study of 9- and 10-year-olds revealed that nearly 50 percent of them exhibited at least one early warning sign of chronic disease. Many pediatricians are now routinely screening for cholesterol levels, high blood pressure, and other early signs of chronic disease. Children identified at risk are treated by dietary modification, for most of these disease states can be controlled, reversed, and prevented by proper diet.

We live at a time when cancer remains one of our most dreaded diseases. Often, we feel helpless to protect ourselves and our children from this invisible threat. Yet, research now clearly implicates diet as a major cause of cancer, accounting for 40 to 60 percent of all cancers. When you consider that cigarette smoking contributes to another 30 percent of all cancers, you begin to realize how much control you do have over the likelihood of cancer striking in your family. In 1982, the National Academy of Sciences made some dietary recommendations aimed at reducing the risk of cancer, and many adults have enthusiastically begun to modify their diets accordingly. However, some well-meaning parents have not realized that some of these recommendations are hazardous to infants and very small children. Babies can not be on low-fat, high-fiber diets without developing some serious health problems. Parents need guidelines for age-appropriate cancer prevention diets, and *The Right Start* gives you these facts.

As parents of newborns, you are universally concerned with providing the best possible care for your infants. With the recent advances in nutritional research, this now includes preventing chronic diseases, such as heart disease and cancer, and extending life expectancy. This is the first baby feeding book to address these issues and to make recommendations on what to do and what not to do. Reading this book may be one of the most important things you can do for your child. We encourage you to integrate these pages into a daily program of good nutrition and to provide your baby with *The Right Start* to a long, healthy, happy life.

Marcia E. and Michael W. Young
Hanover, New Hampshire

HOW TO USE THIS BOOK

The Right Start has been written with you, the busy new parent, in mind. You may not have time to sit down and read every chapter between changing diapers, walking the floor all night, or just trying to maintain order in your life. In fact, you may be lucky to get through one chapter in a sitting. No matter. Though we encourage you to read the whole book, it's not necessary to read it in any particular order. In fact, if you've just brought your new baby home, you may want to start with Chapter 7, Diet of the Nursing Mother, and Chapter 8, Food for the First Six Months. Also, it would be a good idea for you to review the age-appropriate chapters as your baby grows.

The book is organized into three sections. Section I, Food and Health, will give you the basics of nutrition and background on the dietary factors of allergic disease, cancer, heart disease, obesity, and other diseases. For the most part, the information presented is easy to remember and makes a lot of sense. To help you keep all the major points in mind, a summary is included at the end of each chapter. If, from time to time, you forget a few things, chances are a review of the summary will bring the main points back.

Section II, Feeding Guidelines, is designed to give you

practical step-by-step instructions to implement the dietary information you learned in Section I. It will help you establish a comprehensive program of nutrition and disease prevention for your whole family. Individual chapters discuss the specific dietary needs and precautions of the lactating mother and infants from birth through the second year. Charts, tables, and summaries are included for quick and easy reference.

Section III, Foods: Preparation, Recipes, and Suggestions, is basically a cookbook. It will show you how to make your own wholesome and delicious baby food, and give you some helpful suggestions for nutritious family meals and snacks.

The
Right
Start

Section
One

FOOD AND
HEALTH

CHAPTER 1

Basics of
Food and Health

There has never been a better time to apply the old adage "an ounce of prevention is worth a pound of cure." And there is no better time in life than at the beginning! We live in a world characterized by complexity and sophistication. Food is no exception. Every conceivable food is available, year round, at the supermarket—foods that may or may not be beneficial to our bodies. Our environment contains tens of thousands of synthetic chemicals foreign to our biology. In six to eight hours, we can fly from one quadrant of the earth to another and, in so doing, eliminate the natural barriers that have historically helped to control the spread of infectious disease. Our busy and often stressful lives place great demands on our bodies and leave us little time to attend to our basic needs. Never before has man been part of such a complex environment. If we are to live long, healthy, productive lives under these modern circumstances, we must pay close attention to the factors that influence and preserve our health.

As parents in this new world, we want for our children what parents have always wanted for their children—the very best that life has to offer. Yet, we sometimes feel confused and ill-equipped to deal with the problems being generated by our new technologies, problems that often can not be dealt with in the traditional ways we have learned from our own parents.

In the last decade, science has begun to provide answers to the question "How do we protect ourselves from the assaults of our modern society?," and diet is emerging as a significant and controllable factor in promoting health and preventing chronic disease. We now know that what you eat makes a major contribution to your long-term state of health and life expectancy. This encompasses a fundamentally different view of diet and health than in the past, when disease states were usually associated only with severe deficiencies or conditions of starvation. We have begun to recognize that certain components of our diet actually initiate and promote disease and that certain other components can protect us from them. In fact, it can be estimated from the studies of the National Academy of Sciences and the American Heart Association that improper nutrition accounts for at least 75 percent of disease in the United States today. Most significantly, this includes the major killers, heart disease and cancer. By making some simple modifications in your diet, it is now possible for you to significantly influence both the quality and length of your life. This book will provide you with a basic understanding of the dietary factors that contribute to both health and disease and show you how to apply this exciting information to promote the health of your whole family. It will specifically address the special needs of infants and small children, for their requirements are very different from adults.

Although our initial intent is to give you nutritional guidelines for your new baby, it will be obvious that the subsequent suggestions and recommendations are to be applied to the whole family. Your child will eat and do as you do and can do no better than the example set. The side benefit of providing your baby with optimal nutrition will be that you will provide yourself with an increased chance of a healthier life and more years to spend enjoying your children.

Fundamentals of Nutrition

Health depends upon many things including heredity, life-style, personality traits, mental health, and environment. From a perspective of prevention, this book addresses those major aspects of your health that have to do with your diet and the environmental factors that affect the quality of your food supply. Following the guidelines that we present will most probably involve some changes in your diet, all of which are designed to give you and your children the best potential for good health. This first chapter is a basic review of nutrition information, similar to what you were taught in school. It's a good idea to review these topics so that you will better understand future chapters.

Simply stated, we eat to provide for the growth, maintenance, repair, and general functioning of our bodies. Food gives us the energy to fuel our many activities. Food also provides the basic materials from which to build and repair our cells. Food is composed of a large variety of chemicals that are named and classified according to their various properties. The basic chemical components of foods are proteins, carbohydrates, fats, vitamins, and minerals. The goal of sound nutrition is to provide these nutrients in the proper balance, for a most efficient operation of the body.

Let's now look at the various components of food and review their importance in our diet.

Energy

Energy is defined as the power to do work; in the case of the human body, work involves physical and chemical changes. The total of all such reactions is known as metabolism. Bodies need energy to function; they need energy to fuel metabolic processes such as digestion, circulation, tissue synthesis, and repair; they need energy for physical activity and to maintain body temperature. Energy is also needed to support growth in children and pregnant women and to support lactation.

The digestive process breaks down all foods into a form of energy which can be utilized by your body. Each unit of energy is defined by the scientific term, calorie. Different foods provide different amounts of calories. For instance, proteins and carbohydrates provide about 4 calories per gram, whereas fats provide 9 calories per gram. Surplus calories are normally stored as body fat, which is why the important fact to remember about caloric intake is BALANCE. Healthy people who maintain a desirable body weight* for a lifetime have achieved caloric balance. They take in just enough calories in the foods they eat to support the efficient functioning of their bodies. Caloric requirements vary and depend on activity level, body size, age, climate, and rate of growth. For most of us, nature regulates our caloric intake and achieves a state of balance. If, however, you consume a lot of empty calories—that is, foods that are high in calories but low in the basic raw materials needed by your body—you risk upsetting this balance.

*Desirable body weight ranges are published in the RDA and can be found in Appendix B.

Basic Materials

Proteins

Proteins are the basic "stuff" our bodies are made of. They are basic components of all cells, tissue structures, enzymes, and blood components. They are large molecules made from long strings of chemicals called amino acids. Our bodies need proteins, or more specifically, the amino acids, as raw materials from which to synthesize our own body proteins found in cells and tissues. There are 23 different amino acids, and our bodies are capable of synthesizing all but 9 of them. This means that if your diet is deficient in one of the 14 "nonessential" amino acids, your body can synthesize it from other raw materials. The body cannot synthesize the other nine amino acids; therefore, they must be obtained in the diet. They are termed "essential amino acids."

When your body builds a protein, it must have all the necessary amino acids in the appropriate quantities. If an amino acid is not available and your body can not synthesize it, the protein-building process shuts down.

Some foods are called "complete proteins" because they supply all the essential amino acids in the proper amounts. The best sources of complete proteins are meat, fish, eggs, poultry, and milk and milk products.

"Incomplete proteins" are foods that supply some, but not all, the essential amino acids. Typically they are vegetable sources such as beans, peas, cereals, rice, lentils, and corn. These are still valuable protein sources, but they must be consumed in a complementary fashion—that is, they must be eaten in combinations to balance the intake of necessary amino acids. One way to satisfy this requirement is to eat some type of animal protein along with vegetable meals. For instance, milk on your cereal or chicken with your rice. Another way is to team incomplete proteins from vegetable sources up in a way that balances their deficiencies. Many cultures have accomplished this without a scientific knowledge of nutrition by eating grains along with legumes, such as beans or peas, and seeds. A good example is found in Central and South America, where beans are traditionally eaten with corn. But caution should always be exercised when eliminating animal food sources completely from your diet.

Carbohydrates

The principal carbohydrates are sugars, starches, and cellulose. Foods that contain carbohydrates are a major source of energy, vitamins, minerals, and fiber. Such foods are sugar, honey, fruits, vegetables, cereals, baked goods, and milk. Oddly, the human body has no specific dietary requirement for carbohydrate since we are capable of converting proteins and fats into glucose, the simple carbohydrate utilized by the body for energy needs. However, carbohydrates are an essential part of a well-balanced diet. Carbohydrates are a source of dietary fiber. Dietary fiber is the name given to the indigestible part of fruits, vegetables, and grains that adds bulk to the diet and aids in the elimination of waste products.

Some foods containing carbohydrates are better than others. Foods such as whole grains, fruits, vegetables, and milk contain unrefined carbohydrates whose nutritional value is found in the calories, vitamins, minerals, and fiber added to our diet. Other foods that contain simple carbohydrates, mainly in the form of refined sugars, provide a lot of calories, but very little else.

Fats

The word fat is used to describe a number of chemicals not soluble in water. There is no difference between fats and oils, other than the fact that fats are solid at room temperature. Fats are typically found in rich foods of both animal and plant origin. They enhance the flavor and texture of foods, imparting what can best be described as "succulence." For economic reasons, only affluent cultures can afford to have substantial amounts of fat in their diets. High-fat diets and, therefore, the diseases they generate, are found primarily in Western countries. This fact aside, we mustn't forget that we have nutritional requirements for certain amounts and types of fat. In addition to being concentrated sources of calories, fats are essential components of cells and act as carriers for the fat-soluble vitamins, A, D, E, and K. They also prolong the process of digestion in our stomachs, helping us to absorb certain nutrients and creating a "full feeling." Because dietary fats play such a significant role in health and disease, it will be helpful to discuss some chemistry so that you will better understand the complex story of fats.

Dietary fats come in three types: saturated, monounsaturated, and polyunsaturated. This is simply the chemist's way to designate how much hydrogen they contain. Saturated fats carry the maximum number of hydrogen atoms, hence they are "saturated," a situation that also makes them solid at room temperature. Unsaturated fats (mono and poly) contain lesser amounts of hydrogen and are usually liquid at room temperature. All fats are combinations of varying amounts of saturated, monounsaturated, and polyunsaturated substances called fatty acids and hence have different degrees of saturation. Today's technology can make unsaturated fats more solid by adding hydrogen, that is by "hydrogenating." This is done to give a thicker consistency to some foods that are easier to handle as solids. For example, margarines are hydrogenated to make them spreadable at room temperature and peanut butters are hydrogenated to keep them from separating. You must remember that the hydrogenating process makes these fats more saturated.

Our diet must supply us with certain essential polyunsaturated fatty acids unless we are to suffer from a variety of metabolic disturbances. Vegetable oils are rich sources of these nutrients, and it is not necessary to worry about deficiencies. Rather, the problem today is that we eat far too much dietary fat, especially saturated fat. We will discuss the health implications of saturated versus unsaturated fats in greater detail in subsequent chapters.

Vitamins

Vitamins have been the focus of much attention recently and many miraculous claims have been attributed to their use. Some of these claims may be justified while others are exaggerated, and it's time to set a few things straight. Vitamins are nutritional factors that are needed for the body's chemical reactions to take place. They participate in metabolism while attached to other nutrients. That is, they work *with* the food you eat and are not a substitute for a healthy diet. That is why eating vitamins alone will not keep you healthy. Since most vitamins are not manufactured by your body, they must be supplied by your food or by a vitamin supplement. Keep in mind that your body can not distinguish natural vitamins from synthetic ones; consequently, there is no advantage to taking one kind over the other.

Vitamins are classified according to their solubilities in water or fat. As a general rule, any excess of water-soluble vitamins is excreted in the urine, and toxicity is not usually a problem. Vitamins B-3 (niacin) and B-6 (pyridoxine) may be exceptions to this rule, and daily doses that far exceed recommended allowances should be avoided. Fat-soluble vitamins, on the other hand, pose a substantial toxicity threat. These vitamins (A, D, E, and K) are deposited in the tissues of the body (for example, the liver) where they may accumulate to levels greater than that required by the body's metabolism. This can lead to serious metabolic disturbances. By following the recommended daily intake of vitamins and without consuming large amounts of any one food, it is not likely that you will ever suffer the side effects of vitamin toxicities. Children are more susceptible to toxic reactions than adults and can develop toxicity symptoms at relatively lower doses. For this reason, be careful to select an age-appropriate vitamin, and always keep your vitamin supplements under lock and key, as you would any other drug. Eighty percent of all vitamin poisonings involve children.

Table 1.1 lists the 13 vitamins, their dietary sources, and their importance to our bodies.

There is a growing body of scientific evidence indicating that large doses of some vitamins may play a role in disease prevention. In this case, the vitamin may have "super" effects within its normal nutritional role, or it may be involved in some other biochemical process that has the effect of preventing or combatting the disease. This effect of a vitamin is a *pharmacologic* benefit and should be distinguished from its dietary role.

Vitamin C has been the subject of much controversy. This stems mostly from a difference between its nutritional value and its pharmacologic value. Nutritionally, we all need vitamin C to prevent scurvy as well as to maintain healthy connective tissues and to aid in healing. Since our bodies cannot synthesize this vitamin, we must get it from foods such as fresh fruits, especially the citrus fruits, and vegetables.

Pharmacologically, vitamin C presents a confusing picture. While some researchers have reported that the frequency, severity, and duration of the common cold can be significantly reduced by megadoses of vitamin C, others have been unable to confirm these reports. However, there is biochemical evidence that vitamin C is capable of enhancing the immune system by stimulating the production of interferon and other molecules active in fighting infec-

Table 1.1. Vitamins

FAT-SOLUBLE VITAMINS

Vitamin	Source	Function
A (retinol)	orange, dark yellow, and green vegetables, milk, cheese, eggs, fish oils.	required for growth and reproduction, important for healthy eyes and mucous membranes.
D (calciferol)	fortified milk, fatty fish, eggs, butter,	essential in regulating calcium and phosphorus metabolism, hence important for strong bones and teeth.
E (tocopherols)	vegetable oils, whole grains, dark leafy vegetables.	maintains cell membranes, provides protection from chemical toxicants.
K	green, leafy vegetables, fruits, cereals, milk, meats.	essential for normal blood clotting.

WATER-SOLUBLE VITAMINS

Vitamin	Source	Function
C (ascorbic acid)	citrus fruits, other fruits, vegetables.	maintains healthy connective tissue, bones, teeth and gums, aids in healing.
B-1 (thiamin)	yeast, pork, whole grains, poultry, eggs.	needed to convert carbohydrates to energy, essential for healthy nervous and cardiovascular systems.
B-2 (riboflavin)	milk, meat, fish, eggs, yeast,	involved in metabolism of proteins, carbohydrates,

	fruits, vegeta-bles, whole grains.	and fats, essential for healthy eyes and skin.
B-3 (niacin)	meat, milk, poultry, fish, eggs, grains, fruits, vegeta-bles.	needed for energy conver-sion, involved in many metabolic systems.
B-5 (pantothenic acid)	widely available, especially in meats, grains, legumes.	involved in many meta-bolic processes.
B-6 (pyridoxine)	meats, whole grains, vegeta-bles.	involved in many meta-bolic processes.
B-12 (cyanoco-balamin)	meat, fish, shell-fish, poultry, eggs, milk.	essential for healthy red blood cells and a healthy nervous system, involved in many metabolic proc-esses.
Folic acid, folacin	green leafy vegetables, fruits, yeast, liver.	essential for growth and development and a healthy nervous system.
Biotin	yeast, legumes, some vegetables, nuts.	important in metabolism of fats and carbohydrates.

tion. It is also a potent antioxidant capable of protecting against many toxic chemicals and able to block processes that can cause cancer.

A conflict arises for most nutritional biochemists when they consider recommending high doses of vitamin C. Nature seems to have taken elaborate measures to assure that we would not consume such levels. Vitamin C is found in foods at relatively low levels (we would have to eat 33 oranges to get 1 gram of it), and, when we do consume high levels, the body very rapidly excretes it. At prolonged dosages of 2 to 4 grams per day, some adverse effects, including reproductive failure, have been reported. Thus, the controversy over megadosages of vitamin C continues.

Vitamins A and E have also been identified as having disease-preventive activity. This may lead some overzealous health advocates to increase their daily intake of these fat-soluble vitamins beyond safe levels. In the case of vitamin A, excessive intake does have serious consequences. The smart approach is to increase consumption of fruits and vegetables that are high in vitamin A and its precursor, beta-carotene. The body is able to synthesize vitamin A from this precursor. Beta-carotene, which is abundant in orange, dark yellow, and green vegetables and fruits, is the substance that gives these foods their color. Eating too many carrots (too much beta-carotene) can result in the skin taking a yellow coloration, but it does not appear to be harmful.

According to the RDA, vitamin E is relatively safe for adults at daily intakes of 400 IU or less. Children should not be given vitamin E supplementation beyond that found in an age-appropriate multivitamin. It is now well recognized that vitamin E provides protection from various chemical toxicants, such as the atmospheric pollutants ozone and nitrous oxide. It also appears to protect body tissues from oxidative damage, a process implicated in the initiation of cancer, heart disease, and aging. The protective quality of these vitamins will be discussed in greater detail in later chapters.

Folic acid (folacin) is another vitamin of interest because of its importance in growth and development. Folic acid is essential for the synthesis of DNA and RNA, the genetic material, and for the metabolism of amino acids. Thus, a deficiency can lead to impaired protein production as well as aberrations in DNA synthesis. Rapidly growing tissues are the most susceptible to folate deficiency, hence pregnant and lactating women, young infants and adolescents are most at risk. Folic acid is present in green leafy vegetables, fruits, yeast, and liver. It is destroyed by boiling, so canned vegetables and sterilized infant formulas will not be good sources.

Food preparation and storage can adversely affect vitamin potency. Some vitamins are relatively unstable and can be destroyed by high temperatures or prolonged storage at room temperature. Slow defrosting and even excessive mixing or blending can also diminish the vitamin content. Water-soluble vitamins can easily be leached from vegetables as they cook in water. For these reasons, avoid canned or overprocessed foods. Select produce that is crisp and healthy looking and does not appear to have damage from long-term storage. Increase your consumption of raw vegetables, and choose low-temperature cooking methods such as light steaming or quick stir-frying.

Minerals

Minerals are nutritionally important chemicals that are widely distributed in nature. There are 60 minerals found in the body. Table 1.2 includes the more important ones.

Minerals are utilized by the body in complex, interrelated mechanisms. Excessive consumption of one mineral, therefore, may interfere with the absorption of another. For this reason, it is usually best not to take supplements of individual minerals. There are two exceptions that deserve our attention because they are important to proper growth and development and because deficiencies are prevalent. These two minerals are calcium and iron.

Calcium is a major body component. Ninety-nine percent of it is present in the skeleton, where it is held as

Table 1.2. Minerals

Mineral	Source	Function
Calcium	milk, shellfish, some green leafy vegetables.	healthy bones and teeth, vital in controlling nerves and muscles and blood clotting.
Phosphorus	widely available.	important in many biochemical reactions and as a skeletal constituent.
Magnesium	widely available.	essential in many enzyme systems, for proper electrical functioning of nerves and muscles and as a skeletal constituent.
Iron	meats, liver, eggs, vegetables.	needed for healthy red blood cells, involved in oxygen transport mechanisms.
Zinc	meats, liver, seafood, whole grains.	involved in nearly all major chemical reactions in the body, especially important for DNA synthesis.
Iodine	iodized salt, seafood.	important for proper hormonal function.
Copper	shellfish, nuts, liver, whole grains.	important for proper functioning of cardiovascular, nervous and reproductive systems and a healthy skeleton
Manganese	whole grains, vegetables.	essential for protein metabolism, proper growth and reproduction, bone and cartilage formation.
Fluoride	water, meats, vegetables.	strong bones and teeth, reduces dental caries.

Chromium	meats, cheese, yeast, grains.	essential in the metabolism of glucose.
Selenium	seafood, meats, grains.	protects cells against oxidative damage.
Molybdenum	widely available.	essential in functioning of some enzyme systems.

calcium phosphate deposits within a fibrous matrix of bone. Believe it or not, bones are constantly being formed and resorbed, so even a body that has stopped growing has a daily need for calcium. Furthermore, the remaining 1 percent of calcium plays a vital role in controlling nerves and muscles, including the heart muscle, which is why calcium is critical to cardiovascular health. Calcium is also necessary for proper blood clotting. Vitamin D is required for the efficient absorption of calcium, and this is one reason why milk, the primary dietary source of calcium, is usually fortified with vitamin D.

Pregnancy and lactation obviously increase the body's requirements for calcium, which is needed to build the fetal skeleton and to support the growth of the newborn. Growing children need two to four times as much calcium as adults on a weight to weight basis. During pregnancy and lactation and throughout your children's growing years, you should pay particular attention to calcium intakes. If dietary sources do not provide sufficient calcium, a calcium carbonate supplement should be taken. Because calcium is a bulky mineral, ordinary multivitamin tablets do not provide sufficient quantities.

Iron is important for healthy red blood cells and is involved in the transport of oxygen in the body. Iron deficiency anemia is a common condition, most often affecting women. Blood losses during menstruation and childbirth and the increased demands of pregnancy and lactation require additional intakes of iron. Anemia is also common during infancy if maternal iron stores were low, and in childhood during periods of rapid growth. Iron deficiency is characterized by extreme fatigue and a pale skin color.

Body absorption of dietary iron is generally poor and is influenced by body need, the type of iron available, and other factors. Iron available from vegetables or eggs is not as readily absorbed as iron from meat sources. In addition, there are several factors that increase or decrease absorption. For instance, vitamin C enhances the utilization of dietary iron by as much as 250 percent, while antacids and tea interfere with its absorption.

High doses of iron are toxic and can result in organ damage. It is therefore advisable to take a multivitamin with iron supplement and avoid individual iron tablets unless you are under the care of a physician. A cautious note to parents: approximately 2,000 children are poisoned each year by ingesting their parent's iron supplements!

Water and Electrolytes

Water is an essential body constituent, comprising 60 percent of the average adult body. Except under special medical or severe environmental conditions, the nutritional importance of water is not a consideration. For most adults, the requirement of two quarts of liquid daily does not require a conscious effort, because it is a major constituent of all foods and beverages.

The volume of total body water is carefully controlled by an intricate biological system that relies on the concentration of the electrolytes: sodium, potassium, and chloride. These three nutrients are salts which dissolve in body fluids. They regulate fluid retention and blood volume and are important in the control of blood pressure.

Recommended Dietary Allowances

Most information about the nutritional needs of the human body has come from research sponsored by the U.S. National Institutes of Health. This information is updated and published regularly by the National Academy of Sciences in the form of the Recommended Dietary Allowances (RDAs). These allowances are set at levels sufficiently above the minimum daily requirement to assure a healthy functioning of the body and take into account normal variation due to age, sex, body size, level of physical activity, and climate. There are 12 vitamins and minerals for which no RDAs have been established because there is insufficient information on which to base allowances. For these nutrients, Estimated Safe and Adequate Daily Dietary Intakes (ESADDI) have been established.

Appendix A includes the RDA and ESADDI tables providing the nutritional requirements for your family and your baby. This information was included as a reference so that you may check a particular vitamin supplement for completeness or interpret nutritional label information. We have considered the RDAs throughout this book, and all the recommendations made are within these guidelines.

Vitamin Supplements

Historically, some conservative nutritionists have declined to recommend vitamin supplements as essential to good nutrition in the context of a healthy diet. However, as will be explained in later chapters, research has now shown that some vitamins and minerals have disease protective qualities in addition to their basic nutritive value. In this technologic age, it is not always possible to guarantee the integrity of our food supply. Overly processed or inproperly stored fruits and vegetables may have lost most of their vitamins. A multivitamin and mineral supplement may provide an additional degree of health and confidence, and it will do no harm as long as the vitamins are not consumed in excess.

Select a supplement that does not exceed the Recommended Daily Allowance of the fat-soluble vitamins and is within reasonable bounds on other nutrients. A balanced multivitamin and mineral supplement will contain the following:

Table 1.3

RECOMMENDED COMPOSITION OF SUPPLEMENTS

100% of the RDA or ESADDI	vitamins A, D, E, niacin, pantothenic acid, folacin, and iodine.
150% of the RDA	vitamins C, thiamin, riboflavin, B-6, B-12, iron, and zinc.
10–25% of the RDA or ESADDI	calcium, phosphorous, and magnesium.*
50–150% of the ESADDI	copper, manganese, chromium, selenium, and molybdenum.

*Multivitamins cannot supply 100% of the RDA of calcium because this mineral is so bulky the tablet would be too large to swallow. Phosphorous is ubiquitous and is not an essential component of a multivitamin.

A supplement lacking in any of these ingredients or varying greatly from this content should be avoided as it will either be deficient or excessive. As previously mentioned, calcium carbonate supplements can be taken to satisfy calcium requirements. Children should take age-appropriate vitamin supplements. Recommendations are discussed in Section II, Feeding Guidelines.

Basic Food Groups

Nutritionists know that it's difficult, if not impossible, to keep all the varied nutrient requirements in mind when planning family meals. For convenience, the basic food group system was developed to classify foods and simplify nutritional planning. By eating a variety of foods from each of the four basic groups each day, you will be assured of a balanced intake of nutrients. Here are the four basic groups:

GROUP 1. Meats, fish, poultry, and eggs

Animal proteins are excellent sources of complete proteins, providing all the essential amino acids in the appropriate proportions. They are also rich sources of vitamins and minerals.

GROUP 2. Dairy products: milk, cheese, and milk products

Dairy products are also good sources of complete protein as well as carbohydrates, vitamins, and minerals. They are extremely important in meeting calcium requirements.

GROUP 3. Fruits and vegetables

Fruits and vegetables are excellent sources of carbohydrates, vitamins, and minerals, and they add fiber to the diet. Fiber is essential in adults for proper health and disease prevention.

GROUP 4. Whole grain breads, cereals, and flours

Whole grain products add beneficial fiber to the diet as well as an abundance of vitamins, especially the fat-soluble ones, and minerals.

Fundamentals of Your Immune System

Now that you've learned some of the basics of good nutrition, you need to have some understanding of the immune system, your body's defense mechanism against disease. The two go hand in hand in a dynamic relationship that protects you from disease.

Your immune system is a flexible, responsive, and complicated network of specialized cells and biomolecules working in concert to achieve optimal health. This system maintains a delicate balance between your body and the challenges of the environment. The net result is a defense mechanism that repairs damaged tissue, protects against pathogenic (disease-causing) microbes, and prevents cancer by destroying your own abnormal cells.

The immune system is composed of a variety of cell types that circulate throughout the body looking for cellular damage and biological invaders of all sorts. When they find something they recognize as being foreign to your body, they have two modes of attack. They engulf invaders (somewhat like Pac Man), and they secrete a variety of special immune system chemicals that aid in the destruction and removal of these unwanted guests.

Your immune system is able to combat most different disease states. Infections of all sorts are caused by the invasion of living organisms, most of which can not be seen without the aid of a microscope. They are common villains: bacteria such as those that cause strep throat, viruses like the ones that produce the common cold, and all sorts of fungi and parasites. For example, in the case of an infectious disease, such as influenza, the following scenario occurs.

The virus attacks by penetrating your skin through an opening, perhaps through the eyes or through the mucous membranes of the mouth or nose. The virus then attaches itself to a cell and enters the cell (remember that many thousand individual viruses are doing this all at once). The genetic components of the virus (its DNA or RNA) then mix with your cell's DNA (your genetic material) and begin to instruct your cells to make more copies of the virus. The virus multiplies, then spreads to other healthy cells by breaking apart these infected cells.

What does your body do in response to this attack? Some of your lymphoid cells produce antibodies, which are specialized biochemicals that are "educated" to recognize specifically the invading virus. In fact, if you have had the same infection before, these cells "remember" the infection and are therefore able to produce the antibody even faster. The antibody then binds to the virus and inactivates it. Other immune system cells destroy the infected cells and halt the spread of the virus. In this same way, your immune system prevents your body from being overrun by bacterial, parasitic, and fungal infections.

A second, usually more serious type of disease is that termed "metastatic," or cancer. During normal cell growth, your body occasionally makes a mistake and an abnormal cell appears. A properly functioning immune system will recognize this abnormality and destroy it, much the same as it would an infectious agent. If the immune system fails to find and destroy this abnormal cell, the cell can multiply out of control, causing a tumor. One way to insure yourself of optimal surveillance against cancerous cells is to provide your body—hence your immune system—with all the nutrients necessary for its proper functioning. Specific steps to nutritional self-defense against cancer will be discussed in detail in Chapter 3.

There are other disease states that do not appear to specifically involve the immune system, but a poorly functioning immune system may compromise your body's ability to cope with the challenges. These diseases include genetic or inherited disorders, such as cystic fibrosis, physiological, or biochemical disorders, such as diabetes, and the major affliction of Americans today, coronary heart disease, which is caused largely by improper nutrition.

It's easy to envision the benefits you will derive from a healthy immune system. For your children, it may mean fewer days lost to childhood illnesses, common colds, flus, and other infections.

Nutrition and the Immune System

Good nutrition is a major requirement for the development and maintenance of a competent immune system. Numerous studies have demonstrated similarities between malnourished people in developing countries and hospitalized patients in affluent countries. Both groups have compromised immune functions due to improper nutrition; in the former case due to poor diet and in the latter, a disease state preventing normal levels of nutrition. Therefore, proper nutrition is known to be an important component of a healthy immune system. It has also been well established that protein or vitamin deficient diets can suppress immune responsiveness. Most of our knowledge concerning these effects of poor nutrition on immune function has come not from healthy individuals, but from deficiency studies in malnourished animal and human populations.

Immunology has now begun to unravel the complex relationship between the immune, metabolic, nervous, and hormone systems in healthy people. Dietary studies have shown that the level of immune response is related to specific nutrient factors. In fact, some nutrients act directly on cells of the immune system to alter or enhance their capacity to recognize and destroy infectious agents. There is no doubt that your nutrition will directly effect your immune system, and therefore, your health. Presently, there are no definitive, comprehensive dietary recommendations to follow for optimal immune health. However, the guidelines given in this book represent a synthesis of the latest recommendations of leading nutrition researchers. They are formulated to avoid harmful dietary factors and to include those foods which have been identified as having beneficial effects on immune health.

Summary

Now that you have a basic background in nutrition and some understanding of how the body protects itself from disease, you are prepared to go on and look at how your diet affects the development of chronic diseases.

Here is a brief summary of the basics of nutrition:

1. We eat food to provide for the growth, maintenance, repair, and functioning of our bodies. Food supplies us with energy, proteins, carbohydrates, fats, vitamins and minerals.

2. *Energy* fuels our metabolic processes and our physical activities and maintains our body temperature. Energy is measured as calories. Maintaining desirable body weight is dependent on achieving caloric BALANCE.

3. *Proteins* are basic components of our bodies. Proteins are built out of units called amino acids. There are 23 different amino acids. Nine of these amino acids are called "essential" because our bodies can not manufacture them; they must come in our food. "Complete proteins" (meat, fish, eggs, poultry, and milk) provide all of these amino acids. "Incomplete proteins" (beans, peas, cereals, rice, lentils, corn) must be eaten along with some animal protein or in combinations that compensate for their deficiencies.

4. *Carbohydrates* are sugars, starches, and cellulose. They provide energy, vitamins, minerals, and fiber. *Fiber* is that indigestible part of fruits, vegetables, and grains that adds bulk to the diet and aids the elimination of waste products.

5. *Fats* are important sources of energy, essential components of cells and act as carriers for the fat-soluble vitamins. They come in three kinds: saturated, monounsaturated, and polyunsaturated. Our bodies have a requirement for certain essential polyunsaturated fats. These are easily supplied by our diet. Most western cultures have too much fat in their diets and this is the leading cause of chronic disease.

6. *Vitamins* are essential nutritional factors; and they also may protect against some diseases.

7. *Minerals* are essential for normal body functioning and for good strong bones and teeth.

8. Recommended Daily Allowances (RDAs) and Estimated Safe and Adequate Daily Dietary Intakes (ESAD-DIs) are recommendations of nutrient intake prepared by the National Academy of Sciences. They are set sufficiently above the minimum to assure the general population of good health.

9. Eating a wide variety of foods from each of the different food groups is an easy way to assure that your family receives all the essential nutrients in a balanced fashion. The four Basic Food Groups are:
1. Meats, fish, poultry and eggs
2. Dairy products: milk, cheese, and milk products
3. Fruits and vegetables
4. Whole-grain breads, cereals, and flours

10. Good nutrition is essential for the optimal functioning of the immune system.

CHAPTER 1: REFERENCES

1. Committee on Dietary Allowances, *Recommended Dietary Allowances*. 9th ed. Washington: D.C.: National Academy Press, 1980.

2. Suitor, C. *Nutrition: Principles and Application in Health Promotion*. Philadelphia: Lippincott, 1984.

3. *Optimal Nutrition and Disease Prevention: Proceedings of Public Health Nutrition Update, May 1980*. Chapel Hill: Health Sciences Consortium, 1980.

4. The Nutrition Foundation, Inc. *Present Knowledge in Nutrition*. Washington, D.C., 1976.

5. Daniel P. Stites et al., eds., *Basic and Clinical Immunology*. 4th ed. Los Altos: Lange Medical Publications, 1982.

6. Gershwin, M. E.. et al. *Nutrition and Immunity*. Orlando: Academic Press, Inc., 1985.

CHAPTER 2

ALLERGY PREVENTION

Most people do not realize that allergies are one of the most common afflictions in the United States today. And what's more, many allergies are preventable! Allergies are a continuing problem for at least 40 million Americans. In light of the substantial numbers of allergy sufferers and the extent of their discomfort, it's remarkable that so few people understand how to avoid provoking this undesirable condition. The fact is, if parents begin by taking the right preventive steps during their child's first year, the incidence of allergies would be reduced. There are just a few things you need to do in order to help your children be as allergy free as possible, and it's well worth the effort.

There are several different types of allergies, but all represent an inappropriate biological response to a naturally occurring substance. Hay fever and hives are perhaps the most common, but there are other common forms, such as asthma, dermatitis, and food allergies, which for many people produce years of chronic persistent suffering. Chronic suffering is not the only consequence of allergic disease; asthma claims 5000 lives each year.

28

Natural substances known to cause allergic reactions are called *allergens*. Airborne allergens such as pollens, dust, animal danders, and mold spores provoke sneezing, a runny nose, itchy eyes, sinus headache, and lung congestion. Contact allergens such as detergents, chemicals, and fabrics usually cause hives and other types of skin rashes. Allergens in many different foods, such as milk, eggs, corn, wheat, citrus, and berries are capable of provoking a wide range of responses from runny noses and asthma to gastrointestinal distress and headaches.

Medical research has discovered that many allergies have their roots in early infant feeding. Inappropriate or early feeding of some foods increases the risk of developing allergies later in life. In fact, if a baby is a "preemie" and is also fed a cow's milk formula in the first six months of life, most allergists would agree that baby is likely to have allergies as an adult. Even full-term babies can develop allergies from formula feeding or premature introduction of solid foods. This is especially true if there is a history of allergy in the family, for heredity plays an important role in the risk of developing allergies. Table 2.1 shows your child's risk of developing allergies due to inheritance:

Table 2.1.

INHERITANCE OF ALLERGIES

Allergies in Parents	Chance of Your Child Having Allergies
If neither parent has allergies	13%
If one parent has allergies	29%
If both parents have allergies	50–70%

(Source: Data from National Institutes of Health, 1984.)

Infant allergies usually become childhood allergies, which in turn become adult allergies. While it is possible to grow out of the condition, this does not usually happen. In fact, allergy-prone people tend to react allergically to many different substances, and the longer one lives, the more exposure there is to new allergens. Thus allergies usually become lifelong conditions.

For children, allergy symptoms such as a constant runny nose and itchy eyes can interfere with school and play and are annoying for both the child and the family. Furthermore, respiratory congestion often prevents these children from participating in sports and active play, and deprives them of some important childhood social experiences. They are frequently absent from school and may eventually develop behavior problems and have difficulty in concentrating. Asthmatic children are sometimes faced with life-threatening attacks and can spend many hours in hospital emergency rooms. The inability to breathe, even in a mild attack, can be a traumatic experience for a young child, as anyone knows who has comforted a suffering child through a sleepless night. Overall, highly allergic children may suffer not only from the relentless symptoms of allergy, but also from impaired development of physical and social skills.

By now you're probably asking what can be done for the child with allergies. Certainly, with so many sufferers one would think that modern medicine must have an answer. Well, as in most things, prevention is sometimes the only way to provide our children with good health. Allergy treatments take several forms and rarely are 100 percent effective. Treatment is costly, time consuming, and usually must be continued for several years, sometimes throughout life. Unless symptoms are debilitating enough to overcome the obstacles to treatment, many allergy victims prefer to put up with their seasonal discomforts. There are, as yet, no cures. Symptom control, often with unpleasant side effects, is the best one can expect. It obviously makes sense to pay attention to the causes of allergy in infancy, so that you may spare your child a lifetime of compromised health. The information contained in this book, along with your pediatrician's advice, will help you raise your children with the least number of allergies possible.

How do we get allergies, and why is infant feeding so important?

Allergies represent a malfunctioning of the immune system. As we have learned, your immune system protects you from infection by recognizing and destroying foreign substances. Infants are born with incomplete immune systems. This means they are not as able to fight off invading substances such as bacteria or viruses. It also means their immunological responses are sometimes inappropriate when their bodies are challenged by new substances. In the case of allergies, the immune system overreacts to a natural substance that it recognizes as foreign. This sets into action a series of immunological events that establish the allergic response pattern. Once this pattern has been established, chances are it will persist throughout life. As babies grow, they develop more sophisticated immune systems and the capability to handle foreign invaders appropriately. If one can avoid establishing the allergic response pattern in the first year of life, the child may be able to avoid allergies altogether. At the very least, the onset of allergic disease can be postponed and its severity probably reduced.

You cannot develop an allergy to a substance unless you have been exposed to it. Thus, controlling your infant's exposure to allergenic substances while his immune system is developing can protect him from allergic disease. For infants, the most important and controllable of those potentially dangerous substances are foods. In fact, many foods that are usually well tolerated by most adults can be allergenic to children and may set off the child's immune system response.

If you are the one in every five Americans who suffers from allergies, it is quite possible that your allergies were caused, at least in part, by improper feeding in your childhood. Now, through an informed approach to infant feeding, you can make a difference for your child. Even if you don't have allergies, your child still has greater than a one in ten chance of developing an allergy. Anyone can develop an allergy at any age but infants and children are particularly at risk. Infants born in the Northern Hemisphere during May through September are especially vulnerable due to the increased levels of allergenic substances present in the environment during their first months.

It is only within the last ten years that medical research has uncovered the association between infant food allergies and the later development of other allergic conditions such as hay fever and asthma. Consequently, few family practitioners are knowledgeable in providing practical feeding guidelines. This chapter will give you an understanding of food allergies and general guidelines to follow in preventing allergic disease in your baby. Detailed information on introducing foods at the appropriate age will be given in Chapters 8 to 10.

After infancy, children continue to be at higher risk for developing food allergies than older age groups. Knowledge of what foods are potentially allergenic and how to recognize the varied manifestations of food sensitivities will help you avoid problems. This chapter will give you a brief overview of the current state of knowledge. This is a new and somewhat controversial field of medicine which is further complicated by the complexity and diversity of our modern foods. Much research is needed before we can say with certainty how some foods cause illness. However, taking a cautious approach to the use of suspect foods will do no harm and will most likely have a preventive effect.

Allergies in Infancy

Foods are believed to be the cause of just about all allergies in children under the age of one. With an understanding of your baby's developing physiology, an awareness of the symptoms of food allergies, and some knowledge of the allergenic potential of foods, you can bring your baby through this period without provoking his immature immune system. Adopting a cautious attitude and using foods that are low risk (hypoallergenic) is a smart thing to do and takes little effort. Fortunately, as the immune system matures, children usually outgrow their sensitivities to certain foods. This usually occurs by the time they are two years old.

The symptoms of food allergy in infants may surprise you. We have come to accept many as a normal part of infancy. The most common symptoms are digestive and include colic, diarrhea, and spitting up; they may also show up as skin rashes such as eczema and diaper rash. However, an infant food allergy can also be expressed by respiratory symptoms including wheezing, asthma, or chest rattle and nasal congestion with or without a runny nose. These symptoms can make life very uncomfortable for a newborn struggling to adjust to his new environment.

How can we prevent allergies in our babies?

We must remember that human milk is the ideal food for babies. It is not a coincidence that the number of allergic children has increased significantly since 1940 when formulas were substituted for breastmilk and mothers were encouraged to start their babies on solid foods at very young ages. Both formulas and solid foods contain allergenic substances, and very young babies often cannot handle them without undesirable reactions. According to the National Institute of Allergy and Infectious Diseases, an NIH Institute, allergy to breast milk itself is virtually unheard of. However, allergic substances from the mother's diet can enter breast milk and cause allergic reactions in her infant. The likelihood of this happening and how to protect against it are discussed in Chapter 7, Diet of the Nursing Mother.

The following are the most important steps to take in preventing allergies in your infant:

1. Breast-feed! This is the single most important thing to do. Studies show that fewer breast-fed infants develop allergies, both in infancy and in later life. Breast-feeding is not guaranteed to prevent allergies in your infant, but it substantially lowers any risk.

If it is not possible for you to breast-feed and your baby is in a high-risk group for developing allergic disease, it would be wise for you to consult an allergist before you select a formula. Look for one with knowledge of infant food allergies. Your family doctor is a good place to start, but most physicians will refer you to a specialist. Trust your own judgement and continue to seek the proper medical expert until you are convinced you have found one who is listening and will help you avoid allergic disease in your baby. Do this before your baby is born to avoid a last minute rush and perhaps some early feeding mistakes.

Most commercially available formulas are made from cow's milk, and cow's milk is the chief cause of allergies in infants. Even though processing does reduce the allergic potential of cow's milk, a substantial number of infants have adverse reactions to standard formulas. Some formulas are made from soybean milk in an attempt to avoid the allergenicity of cow's milk. However, many infants who are allergic to cow's milk are also allergic to soybean milk.

Soybean formulas are also more expensive. If your baby cannot tolerate these, a physician can prescribe other less allergenic (and more expensive) formulas.

2. If, while you are breast-feeding, your infant acquires one or more symptoms of allergic reaction, review your diet in the preceding days. Did you eat some highly allergenic foods that can pass into breast milk? Consult Chapter 7 for specifics on managing your diet during lactation.

3. Protect your baby from exposure to viruses and environmental allergens such as pollens, animal danders, dust and mold, for at least the first few weeks of life. Do not allow friends or relatives with a cold or flu to visit your baby. Maintain good housekeeping practices to reduce animal danders and dust. If your baby is at high risk, you may want to consider boarding out the family pets for a few months. At the very least, minimize your baby's exposure to animals by keeping them out of doors and well away from his room or bed.

4. The next rule of thumb is to never feed your baby anything other than breast milk (or formula) for at least the first four months. His immune system is simply not prepared to handle other foods. If your baby falls into a high-risk group, it is best to give *only* breast milk for the first 6 months, or longer, as your pediatrician advises.

5. Introduce solid foods slowly and in a systematic manner, as outlined in Chapters 8 and 9. Great care should be taken to give those foods considered to be generally nonallergenic until your baby is old enough to handle something more challenging. If your baby exhibits any signs of food allergy, follow the instructions outlined in Chapter 8.

6. Never give cow's milk or milk products to any baby under six months of age. Cow's milk is highly allergenic and is the primary initiator of allergy in infants. If your baby is at high risk, try to postpone the introduction of fresh cow's milk until he is one year old. Since milk and milk products are an excellent source of protein and calcium in a child's diet, it is important to avoid inducing an allergy to these foods by introducing them before your baby is able to tolerate them. See Chapter 9 for specific instructions on how to introduce cow's milk products.

7. Be very cautious about what you feed your baby when he has diarrhea. When the intestinal wall is irritated, it allows the passage of larger food molecules into the bloodstream. These molecules may be highly allergenic. Your baby is prone to develop an allergy during a bout with diarrhea. Modify his diet at this time to reduce his consumption of challenging foods. Rice, applesauce, and ripe banana may be given to help control diarrhea if he is old enough and has previously demonstrated a tolerance to these foods.

Many parents seem overly anxious to start their infants on solid foods. It's almost as if the ability to handle solid foods is somehow equated with intelligence level. This is simply not so. It is immunological maturity that determines a baby's readiness for solid foods. This process of maturation is naturally programmed and cannot be rushed. Now that you know how important the immune system is in overall health, it's easy to see how a little patience and care at this critical time in your baby's life can have an enormous impact on his future health. Chapters 8 and 9 will guide you safely through this transition period with detailed information on foods that are considered safe and foods that may be hazardous as well as specific instructions to minimize allergic reactions.

Food Allergies After Age One

Millions of Americans suffer from undiagnosed food allergies. The symptoms are so diverse and sometimes so subtle that you may not even be aware that a certain food is causing a bothersome problem (such as recurrent headaches). Many physicians believe that food allergies are the most common cause of our chronic health problems. It is now recognized that many people who were previously labeled as hypochondriacs are actually victims of undiagnosed food allergies. Children are far more susceptible to food reactions than adults and a special awareness is needed to protect them from developing allergies.

Food allergies are also a complicating factor in other allergic conditions such as hay fever (allergic rhinitis). This is because allergic people tend to be sensitive to many different types of substances. If your child does develop an allergy to pollens, dust, or other airborne allergens, the chances are he will also have food allergies, though you may not be aware of them. At the height of "allergy season," his symptoms may be due to a multitude of allergens (pollens, dust, foods) all affecting his body at the same time. The greater the overall challenge to his body, the worse his symptoms will be. If you can reduce the number of substances attacking his body, his symptoms will improve. In fact, there is usually a threshold of tolerance below which there are no symptoms. By carefully controlling your child's ingestion of highly allergenic foods during allergy season, you may be able to substantially reduce his symptoms. Out of season, you may find he still suffers from one of the more subtle symptoms of food allergy.

Table 2.2 reveals some surprising associations between food allergies and some common symptoms.

It is difficult to believe that foods can be the cause of so

Table 2.2.

SYMPTOMS OF FOOD ALLERGIES AFTER INFANCY

General	chronic fatigue, general malaise, sleep disorders
Headaches	migraine, tension, sinus
Respiratory	runny nose, sneezing, sinus problems, asthma, bronchitis, ear infections
Digestive tract	abdominal pain, nausea, vomiting, diarrhea, constipation, gas, bloating, nervous stomach, colitis, rectal itching
Genitourinary	bedwetting in children, vaginal itching, water retention
Bone and joint	arthritis, arthralgia, joint pain, "growing pains" in children
Skin	hives, eczema, unusual rashes, dark circles under the eyes
Behavioral	depression, anxiety, insomnia, hyperactivity of children, difficulty concentrating, moodiness, panic attacks, general behavior problems

many diverse reactions, but you must remember that foods are complex mixtures of hundreds of thousands of different chemicals. It is an extremely difficult task to identify the potentially hazardous components in foods and nearly impossible to predict the variety of reactions individuals might have. Because of this complexity, food allergies are difficult to identify. Although we may not be able to say why a particular food elicits an adverse reaction in some people, we may be able to identify the source of the problem. By learning to recognize high-risk foods and by following a few simple guidelines for food-allergy prevention, you can help your family avoid these troublesome reactions.

Types of Food Allergies

There are three types of "true" food allergies: fixed, cyclic, and masked. These all involve immune response mechanisms. In addition, there are adverse food reactions that do not involve the immune system. These "false" allergies provoke the same symptoms and are thus difficult to distinguish from true allergies. All are most commonly caused by highly allergenic foods (see Table 2.3). A more complete list of potentially allergenic foods is given in Chapter 6. Though these are the foods most often involved in adverse food reactions, there are no completely safe foods. You can develop an allergy to any food, and you are more likely to become allergic to a food that you consume in large quantity.

Table 2.3.

HIGHLY ALLERGENIC FOODS

milk and milk products	pork
egg white	fish
wheat	shellfish
corn	nuts (especially peanuts)
peas	peanut butter
citrus fruits	tomato
yeast	mustard
berries	food coloring
chocolate	

Fixed food allergies generally occur immediately after ingesting a particular food, the reaction is predictable, and usually occurs each time you eat the offending food. For instance, every time you eat strawberries, you break out in hives. It is not difficult to identify this type of allergy, and most people are aware of their problem. Unfortunately, there's not much you can do other than to avoid these foods. In some cases these reactions can be violent and lead to death from shock. An example of this may be an extreme allergy to peanuts, which results in wheezing and labored breathing. On repeated ingestion of peanuts, a severe reaction could occur, resulting in death. If you suspect your child may have such a violent allergy, consult a physician immediately. This is not an allergy to fool around with. Fortunately, this kind of severe reaction is rare.

Cyclic food allergies are more common and are more difficult to identify. Symptoms are often subtle and may not appear for one or two days after eating the offending food. They also may not appear every time you eat that food. In this type of food allergy, the more you eat, the more likely you are to develop an allergy. In fact, you are most likely to become allergic to foods you eat every day. Your body naturally develops a tolerance to these foods, and if you do not exceed your particular tolerance threshold for that food, you will be symptom-free. It is only when you exceed your quota that the allergy appears.

Masked food allergies or "food addiction" allergies are very difficult to identify. Symptoms are less obvious and usually delayed. Consequently, this type of food allergy often goes undetected. In a masked reaction, consumption of the offending food causes your symptoms to immediately improve. You feel better and relate this temporary, good feeling with eating a particular food. When your symptoms return hours or days later, you will unknowingly turn for relief to the very food that is causing your distress. You may even crave this food, which can lead to an increase in food intake and problems of obesity. You are most likely to become addicted to the staples in your diet:

milk, eggs, wheat, corn, sugar. Elimination of these foods may bring on flulike withdrawal symptoms or fatigue, nausea, dizziness, or an unpleasant disposition. Identifying this type of food allergy can be very difficult, yet living with it can have profoundly harmful effects on your health.

No one is born with food allergies, they are all created. With some basic knowledge about food groups and diet recommendations, you can plan family menus that will help you avoid being sensitized by the food you eat. Here are the basic rules for allergies after infancy:

Eating to Avoid Food Allergies

1. Provide your family with a *varied*, well-balanced diet. Food allergies generally arise from an overload of a particular food, exceeding the tolerance level. Therefore, take care to *rotate* the foods you eat. To do this you need to have a general understanding of biological food classifications since foods belonging to the same family are often similar in their allergenic potential. A list of food groups is given in the Appendix D. Try to rotate food groups on a four-day schedule. For instance, if you have pork on Day 1, try not to eat port (or ham, bacon, or sausage) again until Day 4. This will prevent an accumulation of any one food in your body and reduce the likelihood of developing an allergy.

2. Eat foods in moderation. Do not eat large quantities of any one food at one time.

3. Pay particular attention to highly allergenic foods (see Chapter 6 for lists of allergenic foods). These are the foods most often implicated. Remember, there are no safe foods. You can develop an intolerance to any food, and the more you eat of it, the more likely you are to become allergic to it.

These simple rules are not difficult to incorporate into your family meal planning. As you can see from the extent of food allergy symptoms, the benefits of a little extra thought at the planning stage will pay off in a healthier, happier family. Remember, children are much more sensitive than adults to chemicals, both natural and synthetic, in their food and environment.

Cow's Milk Allergy

It is unfortunate that milk and milk products turn out to be among the most highly allergenic foods, for they are an important part of a child's diet. It has been estimated that at least 10 percent of the population is highly allergic to cow's milk. Goat's milk is no less allergenic. The best you can do is to proceed cautiously in introducing milk products to your infant. Chances are, if cow's milk is introduced slowly at an appropriate age, your child will not develop an allergy to milk. If you notice an adverse reaction, discontinue giving milk for at least 60 days and then proceed cautiously to reintroduce. Yogurt and cheese, which are less allergenic than milk, are often well tolerated by milk-allergic individuals. *Because of their extreme allergic potential, consumption of milk and milk products should be kept at moderate levels in people of all ages.*

Another type of adverse reaction to milk is found in people with lactase deficiency. This disorder is most common in North American blacks, most Africans, Greenland Eskimos, and Israeli Arabs. Puerto Ricans and Israelis are also at risk, as well as anyone with chronic bowel problems. Lactase is an intestinal enzyme needed to digest lactose, the primary sugar in milk. A deficiency of this enzyme, which usually develops between age three and puberty, causes symptoms of diarrhea, gas, and abdominal pain on ingestion of milk and some milk products. Again, yogurt and most cheeses can often be tolerated. If you fall

into one of these high-risk groups, you should be alert to
the possibility of your child developing a lactase deficiency.

Treating a Food Allergy

If you suspect that a cyclic or masked food allergy has
already been established, you will probably need the help
of an allergy-trained physician who will put you on an
elimination diet to properly identify the offending foods.
These food allergies may require sophisticated detective
work in order to be pinpointed. You may be allergic to more
than one food, and each may exhibit different symptoms.
After your symptoms have subsided, your physician will
help you challenge your body with various foods until you
have identified the culprits. Thereafter, he will give you a
diet plan, and you may be able to tolerate moderate quantities of these foods if you eat them on a rotational basis.

Diagnosing yourself is probably not wise, unless your
symptoms are well defined and caused by only one food. In
this case, if you are observant and feel you know the
offending food, try eliminating it from your diet. Remember
to eliminate all the foods that may contain your suspect.
Since these foods are often the staples in your diet, you
may have trouble without the aid of a professionally designed elimination diet. Going half-way at this point won't
do. You have to be able to purge your body of this food by
totally abstaining for 60 to 90 days. During this time, if your
hunch was right, your symptoms will improve or go away.
You may then be able to eat moderate quantities of this
food once every four days without provoking your allergic
symptoms.

This chapter is not intended to provide you with all the
information necessary to diagnose your own food allergies.
It is intended to give you a basis for understanding food
allergies, an awareness of commonly allergenic foods, and

general guidelines to follow in planning menus for your
family which will help avoid the problems of food allergies.

Food Additives

Food additives have improved the quality and the
safety of our food supply, yet most of us remain uneasy
about their possible adverse health effects. And for good
reasons. We must realize that it is impossible to predict
with certainty the long-range consequences of adding
chemicals to our foods. Though sophisticated testing can
assure us of an additive's relative safety, we must remember that it is *relative safety*!

Safety depends on how much we eat and for how long;
it depends upon individual susceptibility and upon the
combinations of other foods and chemicals we eat along
with it. The FDA would not approve an additive if it were
shown to have serious adverse health effects. But sometimes, it takes years of accumulating data with large numbers of human guinea pigs to uncover a potentially harmful
effect. For these reasons, the best approach is to eat
simple, basic foods prepared at home and to avoid convenience foods.

When you do buy foods containing additives, check
their ingredients against the lists of additives to avoid given
in Appendix E. There are generally two reasons for concern with food additives: the possibility of provoking an
allergic or adverse food reaction and the possibility of
causing cancer. Additives in the former category usually
cause immediate reactions (within days), which will disap-
pear when the food is no longer consumed. Those in the
later group, obviously, may work silently for years before
manifesting damage. This chapter will discuss additives

that cause adverse food reactions. Additives that are suspected of causing cancer will be discussed in Chapter 3.

Adverse food reactions are most frequently caused by food colorings and some preservatives. When considering whether or not it is wise to consume a particular food additive, you must weight the risks with the benefits. Food colorings add only esthetic value to our foods. Preservatives, on the other hand, have reduced deaths and illnesses caused by food contamination and spoilage. Eliminating food colorings from your diet will not expose you to further risk. This may not be true for food preservatives. The best you can do is avoid the preservatives known to be troublesome.

Table 2.4 presents a list of the more common additives known to cause problems, the foods they are most likely to be associated with, and the usual symptoms they provoke. Remember, that little is known about the allergic potentials of most food additives, so this list may be a partial one.

Food colorings are perhaps the easiest additives to eliminate from your diet. They usually come in packaged sweets and other foods of little nutritive value. Besides being a primary cause of adverse food reactions, many are suspected of causing cancer. Food colorings have long been implicated in behavioral problems of some children, but attempts to prove this relationship in laboratory experiments and research studies have produced conflicting results. For your children's sake, it would be wise to avoid them whenever possible.

Never before have so many chemicals been added to our food supply. New additives are being developed every day. Though we are assured of their safety by their producers, we know there may be hidden dangers. Our best defense is to buy fresh foods or simple frozen foods and prepare them at home. This will avoid the need for food additives and provide our families with an extra measure of protection.

Table 2.4.

FOOD ADDITIVES KNOWN TO CAUSE ALLERGIC REACTIONS

Additive	Common Foods	Symptoms
Colorings:*		
Azo dyes: tartra-zine (FD & C 5), erythrosin, ama-ranth	packaged sweets, cake mixes, soft drinks	asthma, hives, runny nose, head-aches, hyperactiv-ity
Preservatives:		
Sulfites, metabi-sulfites, sulfur dioxide	fruit juices, wine, beer, soda, salads, fresh shrimp, raw vegetables	asthma, runny nose, facial flush, severe shock
BHA/BHT*	oils and fats	asthma, hives
Propylgallate	packaged sweets	asthma, hives
Sodium nitrite*	bacon, ham, hot dogs, cheese	intestinal distress, headaches, hives
Sodium benzoate	soft drinks	asthma, hives, edema, severe shock
Flavorings:		
Monosodium glutamate (MSG)	seasoned salts, dried foods, pack-aged foods, bouil-lons, Oriental foods	facial flush, burn-ing sensation, headache, tingling limbs, palpitations, nausea, sweat, asthma
Quinine	soft drinks	asthma, hives
Menthol	sweets	asthma, hives

Artificial Sweeteners:

| Saccharin* | diet foods | sensitivity to light |
| Aspartame** (NutraSweet) | diet foods | migraines, seizures, panic attacks |

* These additives are also suspected of causing cancer.
**More about the dangers of aspartame in Chapter 5.

Summary

Every day we learn more and more about what we eat and how it affects us. Forty years ago, mothers were encouraged to bottle-feed their infants and to begin solid foods at an early age. This unfortunate advice created many allergic individuals. We now know that some babies are not able to handle the potentially allergenic constituents of infant formulas and solid foods without developing allergies that may persist throughout their lives. If we can avoid provoking this allergic response in infancy, our children will be less likely to develop allergies later in life. Careful infant feeding will pay off in a healthy future.

Food allergies have only recently been implicated in a wide range of symptoms from headaches and runny noses to chronic fatigue and behavioral problems. Though little is known about how certain foods cause these problems, many of the commonly offending foods have been identified. Children are far more susceptible to food allergies than adults. Special awareness is needed to protect them.

Here, in a nutshell, are the simple rules to allergy avoidance:

1. Breast-feed your baby.

2. Introduce hypoallergenic foods slowly at the appropriate age. (See Section II: Feeding Guidelines.)

3. Feed your family a varied diet, and rotate the foods you eat.

4. Avoid eating too much of a possibly allergenic food.

5. Be alert to symptoms of food intolerances.

6. Stay away from food additives.

CHAPTER 2: REFERENCES

1. American Academy of Pediatrics. *Pediatric Nutrition Handbook*. Elk Grove Village, IL, 1985.

2. American Academy of Allergy and Immunology Committee on Adverse Food Reactions. *Adverse Reactions to Foods*. National Institutes of Health Publication No. 84–2442, 1984.

3. "First International Symposium on Prevention of Allergic Diseases." *J. Allergy Clin. Immunol.* 1986. 78; 5:Part 2.

4. Boyles, JH. "Food Allergy: Diagnosis and treatment," *Otolaryngol Clinics of N. Amer.* 1985. 18; 4:761.

5. Editors: Middleton, Elliott, Jr. M.D. et al. *Allergy, Principles and Practice*. Vols. 1 & 2. St. Louis: The C.V. Mosby Company, 1983.

CHAPTER 3

Cancer and Diet

In 1971, President Nixon declared war on cancer, yet today cancer remains one of the most dreaded diseases, accounting for 20 percent of all deaths in the United States. A prodigious research effort has flooded the medical community with scientific information and has provided a better understanding of the disease, yet complete cures are still rare and treatment methods exact a heavy burden from patients and their families. It seems that our best chances for survival is to do whatever is necessary to avoid developing the disease in the first place. A healthy diet can help reduce the risk for yourself and your family of developing this disease. And the earlier you start the better.

Some surprising facts about the causes of many cancers have come out of all this research. The data indicate that as many as 90 percent of all cancers may be a result of life-style and are therefore *preventable*. Diet ranks as the highest risk factor, followed by smoking, alcohol, and occupational and environmental factors. Cancer, like all chronic diseases, develops over time. This means prevention is best when it begins early in life, before unhealthy habits are established and before the disease can gain a foothold. By understanding the nature of some of the dietary factors that may cause cancer you will be able to provide your child and your whole family with the knowledge necessary for a long, happy life.

In 1982, the U.S. National Academy of Sciences (NAS) published its now famous report *Diet, Nutrition, and Cancer*. This 478-page volume reviewed the available scientific and epidemiological information on dietary factors and cancer and formulated a number of Interim Dietary Guidelines aimed at reducing the risk of developing cancer. The Academy concluded that as many as 60 percent of women's cancers and 40 percent of men's cancers may be related to nutritional factors. Furthermore, 30 percent of all cancers are caused by cigarette smoking. So you see, you do have the ability to easily remove yourself and your family from the major threat of cancer. By not smoking and by consuming a diet compatible with these recommended guidelines, you will substantially reduce your risk of developing cancer.

Understanding Cancer

Cancer is a disease in which normal cells become transformed into cells that spontaneously divide in an uncontrolled fashion, usually creating a lump, or a tumor. Often these tumors can spread and invade other body tissues, eventually interfering with the normal functioning of the body. This invasion is known as metastasis. It is important to understand how cancers develop so that we can make the changes in our lives that will prevent the disease from occurring.

Cancers are caused by many different factors in our environment and food supply that continually assault our bodies and result in cellular damage. Although some carcinogens (cancer-causing agents) have always been in our environment and in our food, the complexity of our modern world has so multiplied the variety and the total number of these assaulting substances that we, as biological orga-

nisms, must begin to actively defend ourselves if we are to
survive. Fortunately, nature has also provided us with
certain protective factors, or anticarcinogens. The key to
our self-defense is to add protective features to our diet and
reduce our consumption of high-risk foods.

Scientists now believe that many cancers, the initiation
of heart disease, and the process of aging are all manifestations of the same destructive action caused by "free radicals." Free radicals are ordinary atoms or molecules that
have become highly reactive because they are missing an
electron. They go about trying to make up for this deficiency by stealing electrons from other molecules in our
bodies. In doing so, they damage cellular material. Sometimes this damage is easily repaired by the immune system
and sometimes it leads to precancerous and cancerous
states.

How do free radicals get into our bodies? They come in
the food we eat, in the air we breathe, and in the radiation
we are subjected to, but many free radicals in our bodies
are natural by-products of our own processes of metabolism. So you see, it is impossible to avoid them. That's the
bad news. The good news is that there are many substances
that are "free radical scavengers," that is, substances that
go about deactivating free radicals before they have a
chance to damage our cells. By learning which foods promote cancer (contain free radicals) and which foods protect
against cancer (contain free radical scavengers) we can
readily modify our diet to greatly reduce our risk of developing cancer.

The development of cancer proceeds in two distinct
phases: initiation and promotion. What we have been talking about so far is called *initiation*, an event that causes
damage to our cells. This event is irreversible. Whether or
not this damaged cell will become cancerous depends on
what happens next. The body's first line of defense against
cancer is the immune system. If our immune system is
functioning normally, it will detect damaged cells and dis-

pose of them before they have an opportunity to grow and multiply. Proper functioning of our immune system is, of course, affected by nutrition. We must provide our bodies with all the nutrients and vitamins needed to keep our immune systems operating at peak performance.

If our immune system fails to dispose of this cell, it then enters the promotion phase. If during this time the cell is continually exposed to cancer-promoting agents, it will probably in time become cancerous. However, the good news is that this promotional phase is *reversible*. We can intervene to thwart the promotion of cancer by reducing our consumption of cancer promoters and increasing our consumption of protective factors. In fact, the stage of promotion is most affected by changes in diet.

Another way proper nutrition adds protection is by helping to maintain an ideal body weight. It is estimated that more than 25 percent of all Americans are seriously overweight. Obesity greatly increases our risk of developing cancer as well as all other chronic diseases. Many studies show a direct relationship between total caloric intake and the incidence of several different types of cancers. Since total caloric intake is also highly correlated with a higher intake of total fat, total protein, and animal protein, it is unclear whether or not this increased risk is due to specific components in the diet or simply to an overall increase in total calories. Animal studies have confirmed an increased cancer risk due to obesity and indicate that this risk is reversible if the animal returns to normal or lean weight. Animals on restricted diets develop fewer tumors and have longer life spans. Maintaining ideal body weight places less stress on all body systems and is, therefore, an important goal of good health and disease prevention.

Eating to Avoid Cancer

The great news is that a diet that protects against the initiation and promotion of cancer will also protect against heart disease and may help to retard the aging process. In fact, free-radical damage is suspected in many different disease states. What's more, these dietary guidelines can be easily incorporated into your life-style. No fads, just a well-balanced diet that is low in fat and high in fresh fruits, vegetables, and fiber. This diet can begin to reduce risk of disease at any age, but it is obviously most effective if begun early in life. You can help your baby enjoy a longer, healthier life, if you start now—before the damage is done. (Please see section on cancer prevention in childhood later in this chapter for some important cautions).

There are thousands of different foods that naturally contain mutagens (chemicals capable of causing cellular damage), and research is just beginning to identify these foods and chemicals. Reading the popular articles on the subject can lead us to throw up our arms in despair, for everything we eat, from celery to peanut butter, can cause or contribute to the development of cancer. What are we to do?

We can't eliminate all carcinogens from our foods any more than we can eliminate them totally from our environment. Even if we could, we would still have to contend with those carcinogens produced by our own bodies as we metabolize our foods. What we can do is concentrate on the foods that have been identified as *high risk factors* for the development of cancer. Eliminate those foods from our family meals or, at least, choose to eat them less often so as to reduce the overall challenge to our bodies. We can also add more protective foods to help deactivate the carcinogens we can not avoid. The point is to actively help our bodies fight these invaders and substantially reduce our risk of developing cancer.

Nutritional Risk Factors

Let's look first at the risk factors of certain foods. We need to learn which foods are hazardous so that we may avoid them or at least limit our consumption. However, because many foods contain cancer-causing elements, it's impractical and nutritionally unwise to eliminate all of them from our diets. Instead, we should aim to strike a balance and weigh the nutritional benefits against the risks; this strategy will be easiest to live with and will be the most successful in the long run. Remember, we have ways of defending ourselves in addition to avoiding carcinogens in our foods.

Dietary Fat

Highest on the list of foods that promote cancer is dietary fat. Epidemiologic studies have repeatedly shown an association between dietary fat and cancers of the breast, prostate, and large bowel. In animal studies, high-fat diets have been shown to both initiate and promote cancerous tumors. However, the bulk of data seems to indicate a primary role for dietary fat in the promotional stage of cancer. This is actually good news, for it means that by reducing fat intake, we can prevent a damaged cell from developing into cancer.

Reducing the total fat in your family menus may be the single most important step you can take to prevent cancer in your family. Dietary fat is one of the most significant sources of free radicals in our food supply. In addition, animal fats may contain carcinogenic environmental pollutants. This is because most of these dangerous chemicals are fat-soluble. They can end up in the food chain and are eventually consumed by livestock. Because they are fat-soluble, they are not excreted and are stored in the animal's fat cells.

It is not sufficient to simply substitute polyunsaturated fat for saturated fat. While studies have shown saturated fat to be a more significant carcinogen than unsaturated fat in high-fat diets, they have shown the reverse to be true when total dietary fat has been reduced. According to the NAS report, polyunsaturated fats become the more significant carcinogen in a low-fat diet.

What are we to do? There is no question that the greatest risk is in eating a high-fat diet, whether it is saturated or unsaturated. You must work to reduce your total fat intake, but you must do it wisely. As you will learn in Chapter 4, saturated fat and cholesterol contribute significantly to heart disease, so you will want to reduce these dietary components. (By the way, cholesterol is considered to be a cocarcinogen—that is, it enhances the carcinogenic potential of other substances, so there's another reason to avoid it.) Polyunsaturated fats, while helpful in preventing atherosclerosis, are more carcinogenic than saturated fats because they are far more likely to form free radicals, especially on exposure to heat and light. *Therefore, do not use polyunsaturated oils to fry or sauté.* You can use polyunsaturates in margarine and salad dressing and any other use that will not subject them to high temperatures. Protect polyunsaturated oils from prolonged exposures to heat and light by storing them in the refrigerator.

Now, what will you cook with? Not with "artificially hydrogenated" vegetable oils. These are vegetable shortenings and margarines made from polyunsaturated oils that have been partially saturated to make them solid at room temperature. Research has shown these fats to be even more likely to produce free radicals on heating. Saturated fats (lard, butter) form fewer free radicals on heating, but contribute significantly to atherosclerosis. The best alternative is to use *small* amounts of butter or to use olive oil. Olive oil is a monounsaturated oil; it produces few free radicals when heated and does not appear to promote atherosclerosis. Also avoid all fats that show signs of rancidity because rancid fats have a high concentration of free radicals.

You will have to work hard to reduce the fat content of your menus. The typical American consumes 40 percent of his calories in fat. The National Academy of Sciences recommends reducing this to 30 percent. Unfortunately, we all love fat and are resistant to giving up high-fat foods. Specific recommendations are given in Chapter 6 for ways to significantly reduce fat in cooking and menu planning.

Salt-Cured, Smoked, or Pickled Foods; Nitrates, Nitrites, and Nitrosamines

Populations that consume large amounts of salt-cured or smoked foods have a greater incidence of some cancers, especially those of the esophagus and stomach. Some methods of curing or pickling produce high concentrations of compounds that are known to cause cancer. For these reasons, the National Academy of Sciences recommends that you reduce your consumption of all cured, smoked, or pickled foods. Foods that are smoked and preserved with nitrates or nitrites such as bacon, ham, sausage, cold cuts, etc. add another dimension of risk. While nitrates and nitrites are not carcinogenic in themselves, they have the potential of being converted to a very powerful carcinogen, nitrosamine, in the heat of the frying pan and in the acidic environment of the stomach.

Many people do not realize that nitrates and nitrites occur naturally in a great many foods. Vegetables actually contribute most of the nitrate we ingest. Other sources include nitrate-rich drinking water and fruit juices. Baked goods and cereals account for one third of dietary nitrites. Obviously, we don't want to eliminate these beneficial foods from our diets. The best approach is to counteract them by eating sufficient protective foods that contain free-radical scavengers such as vitamins A or E. These foods will be identified further in Chapter 6.

Molds

Many commonly occurring molds produce toxic chemicals that contaminate our food supply. Many of these are carcinogenic. Among them is a group known as aflatoxins, which frequently contaminate peanuts, corn, and cottonseed and to a lesser extent tree nuts such as almonds, walnuts, pecans, and pistachios. The contamination is greatest in crops grown in the southeastern United States. To give you an idea of the carcinogenic power of this group of toxins, aflatoxin B-1 is classified as *the most powerful carcinogen known*. Epidemiological data confirm a high incidence of liver cancer in parts of Africa and Asia where aflatoxin contamination of food is commonplace. To date, there are no epidemiological studies that directly link cancer in the United States with the contaminated crops, but considering the potency of this toxin, it would be wise to avoid foods that may be contaminated. The National Academy of Sciences recommends that future efforts be directed at minimizing contamination of crops, establishing maximum permissible levels, and monitoring the food supply affected.

Unfortunately, most products do not carry labels telling us whether or not they have been tested for aflatoxins. Health food stores often carry products that are aflatoxin-free. For shopping on the general market, buy premium brands of peanut, corn, and other grain and nut products. Remember, that contaminated crops are more likely to show up in the cheaper, bargain brands because these manufacturers are unwilling to pay the price for quality crops. Avoid cottonseed altogether, for in addition to potential aflatoxin contamination, cottonseed contains a high concentration of another potent carcinogen, glossypol. Avoidance is not always possible since many products (cookies, crackers, baked goods) contain cottonseed oil as an ingredient. This is another good reason to be aware of product ingredients, buy premium products, and bake from scratch.

Other High Risk Foods

As previously mentioned, the list of foods with cancer-promoting potential is long and is constantly growing. Table 3.1 shows other foods identified as containing carcinogens.

Table 3.1.

OTHER FOODS SUSPECTED OR KNOWN TO CONTAIN CANCER-PROMOTING CHEMICALS

Black pepper	Mushrooms
Celery (especially bruised)	Parsley
Parsnips	Alfalfa sprouts
Diseased potatoes	Coffee
Mustard	Sassafras
Horseradish	Figs
Some herbal teas	Alcohol
Chocolate	Fava beans
Cottonseed oil	Rhubarb
Beets	Saccharin
Red dye #40	Orange dye #2
Red dye #32	

Molds on grain, bread, cheese, fruits, apple juice.

Many artificial colorings and flavorings, and food additives from preservatives to emulsifiers and stabilizers (see Appendix E for a more complete listing).

SOURCE: Data from National Academy of Sciences, 1982; and B. Ames, 1983.

Always buy top-quality produce. Diseased or bruised fruits and vegetables generally contain naturally occurring chemicals that are toxic or carcinogenic. These chemicals are produced by the plant in an effort to protect itself from attack by disease or pests. Ironically, it is often healthier to eat produce that has been sprayed with pesticides and fungicides, provided they were properly applied and adequately washed off, than to eat "organically" grown produce that is bruised or has suffered attack from pests.

The risks involved in food additives are often difficult to assess. Many food additives protect our foods from spoilage and contamination, formerly a serious problem that caused much sickness and death. The antioxidant food preservatives, such as BHA and sulfites, are free-radical scavengers and may actually protect us from cancer. They are commonly found in packaged foods that contain fats or oils that may become rancid on storage; items such as cake mixes, baked goods, and dry packaged foods. However, another antioxidant, BHT, has been shown to both promote and inhibit the formation of tumors, depending on the experiment. The truth is that the majority of food additives approved for use have not been tested for their ability to promote cancer. Many are suspected of causing cancer, but it may be years before sufficient information is collected to prove the connection. Saccharin is the only food additive now in use that has been shown by laboratory tests to cause cancer, and it is scheduled to be banned in 1987. Appendix E gives a list of common food additives suspected of causing cancer. This list is likely to grow as more data comes in. The best approach to take is a cautious one. Avoid food additives whenever possible. Foods prepared at home have no need for preservatives, stabilizers, or emulsifiers.

Cooking

The National Academy of Sciences report notes that the cooking of our foods can add substantially to their cancer-promoting potentials. The burnt and browned material produced as foods cook is highly mutagenic, and the longer the food cooks the more carcinogenic it becomes. Any cooking process, such as grilling or frying, that subjects foods to very high temperatures is likely to cause the formation of free radicals. Therefore, take care not to overcook foods. Use low-temperature cooking methods such as steaming, baking, oven-broiling, roasting, stir-frying, simmering, or poaching. Get accustomed to vegetables and other foods that are lightly cooked. These gentler methods of preparation also preserve vitamins, some of which, as we will see, act as cancer-protecting agents. Avoid charcoal broiling, which adds yet another carcinogen to the feast.

Always use a fume hood when cooking. Studies have shown that levels of dangerous air pollutants in home kitchens at dinnertime far exceed the OSHA (Occupational Safety and Health Administration) maximum permissible levels!

Protective Foods

As we have seen, avoiding all cancer-causing agents is not practical or even advisable. What we must do instead is to boost our body's own cancer defense mechanisms. Good nutrition is the key to optimal body functioning, but in addition several specific nutrients have been identified as being cancer-protective. We want to be sure that we consume these nutrients in order to tip the scales in our favor.

Vitamin A

Diets rich in vitamin A, or its precursor beta-carotene, are strongly associated with lower risks of epithelial cancers, specifically cancers of the lung, esophagus, stomach,

CANCER AND DIET   61

intestines, and colon. It has also been demonstrated that patients with epithelial cancers have abnormally low levels of vitamin A in their blood and have consumed diets that are generally low in vitamin A.

In laboratory studies, beta-carotene has been shown to be an extremely effective free-radical scavenger. Beta-carotene is found in dark yellow, orange, and green vegetables and fruits. It is not surprising that the Interim Dietary Guidelines from the National Academy of Sciences emphasize the importance of including an abundant quantity of these foods in our diet.

It must be noted that the data from these studies do not show whether the protective benefit derived from these foods is due to vitamin A, beta-carotene, or some other constituent of these foods. Since high doses of vitamin A are toxic, it is unwise to increase consumption of this vitamin beyond the recommended daily allowance. It is wise to include at least one serving of these fruits and vegetables every day. A table of foods high in vitamin A and beta-carotene is included in Chapter 6.

Vitamin C

Vitamin C (ascorbic acid) is a potent antioxidant or free-radical scavenger. In addition, ascorbic acid has been shown to inhibit the conversion of nitrates and nitrites to nitrosamines. Nitrosamines are those powerful carcinogens that can form in your stomach after eating foods such as bacon and ham. You can actually reduce your risks when eating such cured meats by consuming vitamin C along with your meal, either in the form of a vitamin C-rich fruit or vegetable or in tablet form. The typical amount of vitamin C in an orange is 30 milligrams.

The National Academy of Sciences also indicates that diets high in vitamin C are associated with lowered risks of cancers of the esophagus, stomach, bladder, and colon.

The incidence of stomach cancer in the United States has dramatically decreased now that fresh fruits and vegetables high in vitamin C are available year-round. Conversely, low consumption of citrus fruits has been associated with an increase in gastric cancers.

All this means that you should include citrus fruits, juices, and other fruits and vegetables that are high in vitamin C in your daily diet. These foods provide a valuable source of bulk, complex carbohydrates, and vitamins.

Vitamin E

Vitamin E is another powerful antioxidant. Oxidation is the chemical process by which free radicals are formed. Antioxidants block this chemical reaction. Vitamin E prevents the oxidation of fats and oils to free radicals. A diet rich in vitamin E will help counteract the risks involved in eating fats.

Like vitamin C, vitamin E has also been shown to block the formation of nitrosamines. An important difference between these two vitamins is found in their solubilities. Vitamin C is soluble in water and can be expected to perform its protective functions in the "water-soluble" compartments of your body. Vitamin E is fat-soluble and will protect your cell membranes and fatty tissues from free radical attack. By consuming the maximum RDA quantities of both vitamins, you can provide cancer protection to all parts of your body.

Selenium

Scientific evidence has shown that low selenium intake is associated with leukemia as well as with cancers of the colon, rectum, pancreas, breast, ovary, prostate, bladder, lung, and skin. Low blood levels of selenium are also correlated with cancer death rates. For example, high levels of cancer in a certain section of China have been related to a selenium deficiency in the soil, which produces selenium-deficient plants and animals raised on that soil. When selenium and vitamin E were added to the diets of the inhabitants of the region, statistics recorded a 40 percent decrease in the number of expected cancers.

A large accumulation of data cited in *Diet, Nutrition and Cancer* (NAS), indicate that increased dietary levels of selenium protect against a variety of cancers. Selenium consumed at RDA levels appears to protect cell membranes from free radical attack and is especially effective against polyunsaturated fats.

Selenium also has the ability to protect against heavy metal toxicity. It appears to detoxify metals such as cadmium and mercury and protect against their carcinogenic effects.

To assure adequate selenium intake, it is prudent to select a multivitamin preparation that contains selenium, but do not take more than 200 μg/day which is the maximum RDA. High levels of selenium are toxic and have been associated with serious birth defects. *Supplemental dietary selenium is not recommended for pregnant women or for children under age 4.*

Fiber

Cancer and many other chronic diseases are associated with low dietary fiber. Cancers of the colon and rectum have increased substantially since the early 1900s when superrefined white flour was introduced, with a subsequent reduction in whole-grain flours. In fact, colorectal cancer is the number two cancer killer. This same cancer is rare in cultures with high-fiber diets.

Foods that are high in fiber are vegetables, fruits, and whole-grain cereals. They contribute indigestible food fibers that create bulk in the intestines. This bulk protects the intestinal wall from intimate and prolonged contact with carcinogens. Bulk also hastens the elimination of foods; thus carcinogens have less time to damage healthy cells.

In addition to adding abundant amounts of fresh fruits and vegetables to our diets, we must also concentrate on getting sufficient quantities of legumes (beans and peas) and whole grains. Serve more whole-grain cereals and breads, bran, granola, oats, etc. and avoid overprocessed refined baked goods. It is best to obtain fiber from dietary sources and avoid fadlike supplements. Caution: As with all dietary factors, balance is key. Too much fiber in the diet can provoke health problems. This is especially true for children under age two. Please refer to specific recommendations in Section II.

A high-fat diet in combination with a low-fiber intake appears to carry the highest associated risk of cancer.

Cruciferous vegetables

The Committee on Diet, Nutrition and Cancer recommends adding adequate quantities of cruciferous vegetables (those belonging to the mustard family) to your diet because they have been found to inhibit carcinogenesis. This means that you should include cabbage, Brussels sprouts, broccoli, and cauliflower in your meals two to three times per week.

Cancer Prevention in Childhood: Some Cautions

The sooner you begin a diet aimed at reducing cancer risk, the more likely you are to be successful at avoiding the disease. However, not all recommendations for adults can be applied to infant feeding. Pediatricians are beginning to see babies who have stopped growing, fail to thrive, or have severe intestinal disturbances due to diet. It seems their parents, in a well-intended attempt to minimize future disease risk, have put them on low-fat, high-fiber diets. By the time your child is two years old, he can be eased into a complete disease-prevention diet. But, in the meantime, follow these rules:

1. *Do not aim for a high-fiber diet.* Infants have high caloric requirements to support their enormous growth. They also have small stomachs. A high-fiber diet would provide a lot of bulk and very few calories. Fiber is also too rough for immature intestines and can cause considerable distress. Do not be concerned about adding fiber until your child is two years old.

2. *Do not feed low-fat dairy products.* Breast milk has a high fat content, especially saturated fat. These are calories your baby needs. When adding cow's milk to his diet, give him whole milk (3 percent fat). In addition to having more calories, it is easier for him to digest. Low-fat milk and skim milk have too many solids for your baby's kidneys to handle before the age of two.

3. *Select lean meats.* As with the family's diet, select lean cuts of meat for making baby food. Trim all fat before cooking, and skim fat after cooking.

4. *Cook foods lightly.* To prevent build-up of carcinogens and to preserve vitamins, steam or microwave all fruits, vegetables, and meats *lightly.*

5. *Avoid foods known to contain carcinogens, feed foods high in protective factors.* Serve your baby dark yellow, orange, and green fruits and vegetables. Avoid all suspect foods, including additives, colorings, and preservatives.

6. *Give your baby an age-appropriate multivitamin each day.* See Section II for more specific information. Do not

give a selenium-containing multivitamin to children under 4 years old.

Summary

Simple diet recommendations have come out of the National Academy of Science's *Diet, Nutrition and Cancer* report. By incorporating these suggestions into your family menus, you can reduce risk of developing cancer by 40 to 60 percent. By not smoking, you can eliminate an additional 30 percent risk of cancer, thus reducing your overall probability of getting cancer by as much as 90 percent. Here are the rules to follow:

1. Reduce your consumption of high-risk foods.

* Reduce *total* dietary fat to less than 30 percent of your total caloric intake. For a 2000-calorie diet, this is about sixty-seven grams of fat. Another way to view this, is to eliminate 25 percent of the fat from your diet.

* Limit your consumption of salt-cured, smoked, and pickled foods.

* Avoid food additives, colorings, and flavorings.

* Be aware of the foods known or suspected of promoting cancer, and weigh the benefits with the risks.

2. Increase your consumption of protective factors.

* Eat plenty of dark yellow, orange, and green fruits and vegetables.

* Eat plenty of cruciferous vegetables such as cabbage, Brussels sprouts, broccoli, and cauliflower.

* Add fiber in the form of whole-grain breads and cereals such as bran, whole wheat, oats, granola, etc.

* To assure adequate consumption of the protective

vitamins A, C, and E, take an age-appropriate multivitamin each day. For adults, this should include selenium.

3. Ease your baby into a cancer-preventing diet *after* his second birthday.

4. Remember that experimental research is ongoing and that new information concerning the relationship between foods and cancer will continue to surface. Try to keep up on new developments by reading nutrition articles in newspapers and magazines. Be alert to authoritative medical reports on radio or TV. By actively listening and learning, you will best benefit from the flow of new information.

CHAPTER 3: REFERENCES

1. Committee on Diet, Nutrition, and Cancer, National Academy of Sciences. *Diet, Nutrition, and Cancer.* Washington, D.C.: National Academy Press, 1982.

2. Ames, B. "Dietary Carcinogens and Anti-carcinogens: Oxygen free radicals and degenerative diseases." *Science. 1983.* 221:1256–1264.

3. American Academy of Pediatrics. *Pediatric Nutrition Handbook.* Elk Grove Village, IL, 1985.

4. National Heart, Blood and Lung Institute. *Symposium on Oxygen Free Radicals. 1986.* In press.

5. Hausman, P. *Foods That Fight Cancer.* New York: Rawson Associates, 1984.

CHAPTER 4

A Healthy Heart

Cancer is not the only chronic disease that may have a strong nutritional component. In fact, chronic diseases, by their very nature, develop slowly over a long period of time and are greatly influenced by the way we feed our bodies. Chronic diseases are also among the most difficult to treat successfully. This is because damage to vital body systems is usually severe and often irreversible. Medical science is now coming to accept some harsh realities concerning our ability to cure people once they become chronically ill. But we are also discovering how simple it is to dramatically lower the risk of these diseases, if we start early enough. The next decade will see a new era in medicine where prevention is foremost in the minds of physicians, for we now know that this is the most sensible approach to disease control.

Heart disease, stroke, and related disorders of the cardiovascular system top the list of diseases caused by dietary factors. This group of diseases is the number one killer in the United States today, accounting for nearly 50 percent of all deaths. More than 63 million people suffer from some form of these deadly diseases. Many die suddenly of a heart attack at relatively young ages without any forewarning of their condition. Though we are accustomed to think of heart disease as an affliction of aging, physicians are now beginning to consider it a pediatric disease. There is compelling evidence that cardiovascular disease begins very early in life.

The behavior patterns that increase risk of coronary heart disease (CHD) are established in childhood and precipitate early physiological changes. If we are to conquer CHD, we must start with our babies. Atherosclerosis, hardening of the arteries, is the major cause of heart disease and related disorders. More and more clinical evidence is revealing early signs of atherosclerosis in very young children. Autopsies of apparently healthy young men from the Korean War and the Vietnam War revealed the presence of atherosclerotic lesions in 70 percent of them, and 40 percent had severe occlusive lesions! These conditions did not develop overnight. More recently, autopsies of healthy children have demonstrated a direct relationship between blood cholesterol levels and physical evidence of atherosclerosis. It is clear that the causative factors are active early in life.

Many pediatricians now recommend routine screening of cholesterol levels. This can be done with a simple blood test, often using just a finger-prick of blood. American children have higher cholesterol levels than other populations, and these levels tend to rise over time. A child with a blood cholesterol level greater than 185 mg/dl would be considered at high risk for developing atherosclerosis. In the majority of these cases, *diet* is the primary cause. Early detection of the condition combined with dietary modification can protect these children from future disease—before their bodies have been damaged.

What Causes Atherosclerosis?

Atherosclerosis is a chronic condition in which plaques, or fatty deposits, build up on the inside walls of your arteries, causing them to narrow and become inflexible. As this condition progresses, it becomes more and more difficult for your heart to pump blood through these constricted channels. This causes your heart to work harder, and it raises your blood pressure. Eventually, a clot may get trapped in the constricted area, cutting off the supply of blood to your heart or your brain. If this blockage occurs in the coronary artery, the result is a heart attack; if it occurs in an artery in the neck or brain, the result is a stroke.

How do you get atherosclerosis? There seems to be a genetic factor to this disease. That is, if your family has a history of early heart disease, you are at greater risk, but the degree of this risk is dependent on other variables as well. These other factors include high-fat diets, cigarette smoking, high blood pressure, male sex, diabetes, obesity, and a sedentary life-style. This is actually good news, for most of these risk factors are within your control. The dietary factor is so clear that a good preventive diet can do wonders to reduce even the highest risk. Conversely, a life-style and diet that raise blood cholesterol levels can provoke atherosclerosis in people with no family history of heart disease. The American life-style of a rich diet combined with a reduced rate of physical exercise is responsible for the high rate of coronary heart disease in this country, one of the highest in the world. Look at the statistics. In the United States, the male death rate due to CHD is 100 deaths for every 100,000 people. In Thailand, where people eat a very low-fat diet, this rate drops to 0.5 deaths, whereas in France, a country with a moderate fat diet, the rate is 30 deaths per 100,000.

Plaque Formation

The atherosclerotic process begins with an injury to the wall of an artery. In response to this injury, your immune system sends special cells to the area to begin the healing process. Some of these cells, however, release potent growth factors that stimulate the growth of muscle cells. The growth of these cells results in a ragged or bumpy patch on the interior artery wall. Thereafter, as blood is pumped past this spot, some components, specifically fats and cholesterol, get caught up on the ragged area and stick to it. As the body battles this situation, scavenger cells arrive to try to digest the fats away, adding to the accumulating debris. Finally, to stop this progression, the body caps it all off with scar tissue, and a mature plaque is formed. The result is a narrowed and less flexible artery. This process usually proceeds over a span of 30 to 40 years. However, the rate of plaque formation is governed by diet and genetics. In high-risk individuals, plaque formation can be greatly accelerated by a number of factors, including a high-fat diet.

Diet and Atherosclerosis

Dietary intervention at any point in this scenario can retard or even reverse the atherosclerotic process. It is now believed that the initial injury to the arterial wall may be caused by our old friends, the free radicals. These are the same chemicals that cause some cancers by damaging our cellular material. As you will remember from Chapter 3, fats are the single greatest source of free radicals in our diet, so you can minimize this initial injury by reducing the fats in your diet. You will also remember that free radicals can be defeated by adding "free radical scavengers" to your diet. Thus the same diet that will help prevent cancer will also help to prevent cardiovascular disease.

But that's just the beginning of this story. Once the arterial damage has occurred, it is the saturated fats and cholesterol in our diets that begin the plaque formation. Studies in animals show that severe atherosclerotic lesions can be induced quickly with a diet high in saturated fats. But more important, there are no examples of human populations developing atherosclerosis without also having hyperlipidemia—too much fat in the blood. In other words, atherosclerosis does not happen to people with normal blood cholesterol levels. There is no incidence of athero- sclerosis in people with blood cholesterol levels of 150 milligrams per deciliter (mg/dl) or less. A slight risk extends to people with levels up to 200 mg/dl, and above this level risk increases significantly with increasing cholesterol lev- els. To find out your risk of developing atherosclerosis, have your physician order a blood cholesterol test. Most routine adult exams include this measurement, but many pediatric check-ups do not. If you are concerned about your child's cholesterol, discuss this with your pediatri- cian.

It is important to make the distinction here between dietary cholesterol and blood cholesterol. Dietary choles- terol is usually found along with animal fats in such foods as eggs, dairy products, and meats. When you eat dietary cholesterol, it does not go directly to your bloodstream to raise your blood cholesterol. It goes to your liver to be processed. Depending on body needs, it is then sent out to cells requiring cholesterol, or it is excreted. This system works quite well unless your diet is high in cholesterol and saturated fats.

As with most questions of human chemistry, the pic- ture is not as simple as it initially appears. Cholesterol and other fatty substances called lipids are transported through your bloodstream by molecules called lipoproteins. It turns out there are "good" lipoproteins and "bad" lipoproteins. The former, called HDL (High Density Lipoprotein), helps to remove excess cholesterol from your blood and actually protects against heart disease. If your total blood choles- terol has more of this "good" cholesterol, your risk is reduced. The "bad" lipoprotein is called LDL (Low Den- sity Lipoprotein). This molecule carries cholesterol through your system, depositing the excess in arterial plaques. The higher your level of LDL cholesterol, the higher your risk of cardiovascular disease. This is why physicians now test for both HDL and LDL cholesterol, often as a follow-up study if your total cholesterol is borderline or high.

Now, back to dietary cholesterol. *If you eat a low-fat diet*, the cholesterol you consume probably has little effect on your blood cholesterol level. Your liver compensates for varying levels of dietary cholesterol and maintains a normal blood level. However, approximately 20 to 30 percent of the U.S. population is genetically hypersensitive to cholesterol. That is, consumption of cholesterol for these individuals does result in an elevation of their blood cholesterol levels. For these people, extreme dietary measures and special medication may be necessary to control blood cholesterol levels. For the rest of us, it is the excess fat we consume that upsets our body's ability to maintain normal blood cholesterol levels.

The story of dietary fats is really a complicated one. Not all fats have the same effect on our blood cholesterol levels. Generally speaking, saturated fats and cholesterol (they are two different things) raise blood cholesterol levels; monounsaturated fats are neutral; and polyunsaturated fats lower blood cholesterol levels. Many people do not realize that all dietary fats contain varying degrees of saturation—they are combinations of saturated, monounsaturated, and polyunsaturated fats. The more saturated they are, the more solid they will be at room temperature; the more polyunsaturated they are, the more liquid they will be. This fact gives you a general guideline to go by, but there are some exceptions to this rule, so it's better to know what foods to avoid and what foods to add to your diet.

In addition, you should understand that when a food label says "hydrogenated" that is another way of saying "saturated." Many foods start out with polyunsaturated oils, which are then hydrogenated (hydrogen is added) and they become saturated or partially saturated. Margarines are a perfect example. If they were not hydrogenated, most of them would not form a spread at room temperature. The harder the margarine, the more saturated it is. In fact, some margarines are not much healthier to eat than butter. Read the ingredient labels. Avoid the inexpensive brands made from palm or coconut oils. Select instead margarines made from safflower, sunflower, or corn oil. Also remember that cholesterol and saturated fat are two different entities. Vegetable shortenings very proudly claim to be "cholesterol free," but they are surely high in saturated fats.

Then there are some oils that will fool you. For instance, coconut oil and peanut oil are unusually powerful promoters of atherosclerosis. They are used experimentally to induce plaques in laboratory animals. It's a good idea to avoid these oils whenever possible. Unfortunately, the food industry uses the relatively inexpensive coconut oil as a standard ingredient in baked goods and other products.

Table 4.1 includes a list of foods to avoid to lower your risk of coronary heart disease. In general, saturated fats such as those found in meat, cheese, and butter raise blood cholesterol levels and contribute to plaque formation.

Polyunsaturated fats, as found in most oils of vegetable origin, actually appear to reduce cholesterol production somewhat and possibly aid in its breakdown. They help to reduce your levels of LDL (bad) cholesterol, but they also reduce your levels of HDL (good) cholesterol. It's a good idea to substitute polyunsaturated fats for the saturated ones discussed. Table 4.2 lists the most common polyunsaturated oils and spreads, ranking them according to their degree of polyunsaturation. Try to use the oils and margarines with the highest degree of polyunsaturation. As you substitute these fats for the more saturated ones in your diet, you must keep one thing in mind. We learned in Chapter 3 that polyunsaturated fats are more likely to form free radicals on heating, thereby enhancing our risk of developing cancer. Don't use them in frying or sautéing

Table 4.1.

FOODS THAT INCREASE RISK OF ATHEROSCLEROSIS

peanut oil	coconut oil
palm oil	butter
cocoa butter	shortening
lard	beef tallow
beef	bacon
pork	ham
fried foods	poultry (dark meat)
sausage	organ meats
whole milk	high-fat cheeses*
egg yolk	ice cream
cream	avocado
chocolate	coconut
peanut butter	oysters

*Examples of high-fat cheeses: Brie, Camembert, cream cheese, creamed cottage cheese, American, Jack, Swiss, bleu, and cheddar.

where they will be subjected to high heat, and always store them in the refrigerator. Use monounsaturated (neutral) olive oil for high-temperature cooking. It's less likely to form free radicals, and it does not raise blood cholesterol levels.

There are even fats that can substantially lower blood cholesterol and *protect* against atherosclerosis. These are the Omega 3 oils found in high concentrations in some of the more oily fish. Like other polyunsaturated fats, they have been shown to reduce LDL (bad) cholesterol levels, but more important, they do not lower HDL (good) cholesterol levels. They also prevent clot formation and reduce the likelihood of fats adhering to an arterial plaque. Diets rich in Omega 3 oils have been shown to retard and even reverse the atherosclerotic process. This seems to be the reason why Eskimos, who eat a diet very high in fats, have such low incidence of heart disease. Studies have shown that as

Table 4.2.

POLYUNSATURATED FATS

Oils:	% polyunsaturation
safflower oil	74
sunflower oil	66
wheat germ oil	62
corn oil	59
soybean oil	58

Margarines:	
safflower (tub margarine)	60
corn (tub margarine)	48
corn, soybean, cottonseed (stick margarine)	28

Mayonnaise:	
soybean	52

Table 4.3.

FISH HIGH IN OMEGA 3 OILS

salmon	herring
swordfish	tuna
snapper	mackerel
sardines	trout*
pompano	lake whitefish*

*Remember that freshwater fish are more likely to contain industrial pollutants than ocean fish. For this reason, unless you're sure of the purity of the source, limit your consumption.

little as two small meals of these fish per week can significantly lower the risk of coronary heart disease. This is probably one of the simplest and best things you can do to prevent heart disease in your family.

Recently, pharmaceutical companies have begun to market fish oil concentrates high in Omega 3 oils for use as dietary supplements in the prevention of coronary heart disease. If you are at high risk for CHD, these supplements may be of benefit to you. For your children, a well-balanced low-fat diet that includes ample fish dishes may prevent them from ever needing such a supplement.

Other Dietary Factors in Atherosclerosis

While dietary fat is the most significant nutritional factor influencing the development of atherosclerosis, other food components have been identified that promote or protect against this disease. For example, unrefined carbohydrates (high in dietary fiber) appear to be less atherogenic than the simple sugars found in highly refined food products. Water-soluble dietary fiber, such as found in fresh fruits and vegetables (specifically, the legume family of beans and peas, apple pectin, and oat bran) alters cholesterol metabolism and lowers risk of atherosclerosis, whereas the water-insoluble forms (found in the fibers of vegetables and grains) have no effect. Recently, several mineral deficiencies have been implicated in the promotion of experimental atherosclerosis. These include deficiencies of magnesium, copper, vanadium, and chromium. While the significance of this discovery for humans is not yet known, a nutritious and balanced diet, supplemented with a good vitamin and mineral preparation, will protect you from such deficiencies.

Other Risk Factors of Cardiovascular Disease

Atherosclerosis is the major risk factor of coronary heart disease. However, there are other factors influencing its development over which you have control. These include high blood pressure, obesity, cigarette smoking, and lack of exercise. The causes of high blood pressure and obesity and the preventive measures you can take to avoid them are discussed in Chapter 5.

In this day and age, it seems ridiculous to have to say anything more on the evils of cigarette smoking, yet many otherwise sensible people are still not getting the message. What is even more distressing are the *parents* who continue to smoke with small children in the house. As mentioned earlier, children are far more susceptible to the pollutants and chemicals in our environment. The truth about cigarettes is this: they suppress your immune system, raise your blood pressure, and deliver high concentrations of free radicals directly into the delicate and vulnerable tissues of your lungs. In addition, they directly inhibit your body's ability to deactivate free radicals. It is not just the risk of lung cancer that is increased with cigarette use. It is the risk of *all* disease. Your immune system is your most valuable ally. You should never risk compromising its ability to defend your body from attack. For your children, passive smoking is a real hazard. Studies conducted by the National Institute of Environmental Health Sciences indicate that your child's lifetime risk of developing leukemia increases by 70 percent if he resides in a household with one smoker and by 460 percent with two smokers. In 1986, the U.S. Surgeon General, acting upon what he believed to be overwhelming evidence of the dangers of inhaling other people's cigarette smoke, began a campaign to protect the rights of nonsmokers. Much like the warnings of his predecessor in the 1950s linking cigarette smoking with cancer and heart disease, these warnings are being met with resistance and public skepticism. As evidence accumulates, public opinion will change. Meanwhile, if you love your child, you will protect him from passive smoking.

Regular daily exercise is another preventive method that works not just for coronary heart disease, but for all diseases. Your whole body and your immune system work better if you lead a physically active life. Statistics show that some populations who eat high fat diets have a lower incidence of heart disease because they exercise more than Americans. Perhaps this is because blood cholesterol measurements record a decrease in LDL (bad) cholesterol and an increase in HDL (good) cholesterol with physical activity. The proof is there; exercise works! And studies show that a brisk two mile walk three times a week is probably sufficient for most people.

Fast Foods

Perhaps the greatest threat to our children's good health is the current passion for fast foods. In persuasive advertising campaigns, children are lured into fast-food restaurants with promises of giveaways, parties, and fun. Most are outfitted with playgrounds and other enticements. Yet, how many of us are aware of the fact that fast-food chains are primary contributors to future cancer, atherosclerosis, and obesity in our children.

Fast fast food responsible for 20 percent of all the fat added to our food, and fast-food restaurants serve a staggering 20 percent of the population daily. Virtually all their entrees are fried, and, what's more, they are often fried in beef tallow, a fat that is both saturated and high in cholesterol. A typical meal can easily contain the maximum recommended daily fat intake, all at one sitting. Even their fish and chicken meals are fried, turning healthful food into disease-provoking fare.

Beef tallow, a commercial form of lard made from beef fat, has been the fat of choice for two reasons; economy and taste. This is the secret, succulent ingredient that creates fast-food addicts. Food chains have been unwilling to substitute other more healthful fats out of fear of losing customers who crave this taste.

Lately, there have been campaigns by some of these companies to improve their health image. Now, they are advertising products "cooked in vegetable oil." But unless they tell you what kind of vegetable oil, this change may not improve the "health" of their food. The inexpensive oils, coconut and palm, are highly saturated. And, of course, any vegetable oil can be turned into a saturated fat by hydrogenation. In addition, high-temperature frying causes the formation of free radicals. Our objective, moreover, is to reduce the *total* fat in our diets. There's no way you're going to succeed at this and continue to eat at fast-food restaurants. If you are serious about disease prevention you can not allow your children to develop these dangerous habits. Choose, instead, one of the many family-style restaurants that offer menus with basic sandwiches such as tuna fish and sliced chicken, salads, soups, etc., and stay away from fried foods.

Summary

Cardiovascular disease is the number one killer in the United States today, but it needn't be. Many of the identified risk factors are completely within your control. By making sensible modifications to your diet and your lifestyle, you can substantially reduce the risk to yourself and your family. Your children stand to gain the most from this approach, for their young, healthy bodies have not yet been damaged by years of poor eating habits.

Here are the guidelines to follow in preventing cardio-vascular disease:

1. Eat a low-fat diet. Both cancer and heart disease have their roots in a high-fat diet. The average American consumes 40 percent of his daily calories in fat. It is recommended that this figure be reduced to 30 percent. Babies should be introduced *gradually* to a low-fat diet after they reach their second birthday. *Do not feed infants a low-fat diet*. Growth and development can be severely compromised when babies are fed low-fat diets. Please refer to Section II for specifics.

2. Restrict your intake of saturated fats and choles-terol, substituting polyunsaturated fats wherever possible, except for high-temperature cooking. Fry with olive oil or small amounts of butter. Avoid peanut oil and coconut oil altogether.

3. Eat more fish, especially those fish high in Omega 3 oils. Just one or two small servings per week can substan-tially reduce the risk of your family developing heart dis-ease.

4. Add fiber to your diet. The fibers found in fresh fruits and vegetables appear to aid in the excretion of cholesterol. Again, remember not to start your baby on a high-fiber diet until after his second birthday.

5. Do not smoke cigarettes.

6. Maintain normal body weight.

7. Keep your blood pressure under control.

8. Exercise regularly.

CHAPTER 4: REFERENCES

1. American Academy of Pediatrics. *Pediatric Nutrition Handbook*. Elk Grove Village, IL., 1985.

2. Robert I. Levy, M.D., Chairman. *Primary Prevention of Atherosclerosis in Childhood: The Role of Lipids*. Proceedings from a videoconference. New York: Biomedical Information Corporation, 1985.

3. Davidson, M. H., and Liebsonn, P. R. "Marine Lipids and Atherosclerosis: A Review," *Cardiovascular Reviews & Reports. 1986. 7;* 5:461–472.

4. The American Heart Association. *1986 Heart Facts*. Dallas, TX, 1986.

5. Goodman-Malamuth, L. "Ad Nauseum: The McDonaldization of Childhood." *Nutrition Action Health Letter* Center for Science in the Public Interest. 1986. 13; 3:1.

CHAPTER 5

Obesity, Hypertension, and Other Ailments

Obesity

Obesity has been identified by the American Academy of Pediatrics as the most important nutritional disorder in the United States today. In addition to increasing our risk of developing chronic diseases (cancer, heart disease, stroke, atherosclerosis, hypertension, and diabetes), obesity can have profound psychological consequences, especially on the social adjustments of children. We would all like to spare our children the burden of being overweight, and it is crucial that we begin now. Studies have shown that long-term success in treating obesity is rare and prevention may hold the only hope for conquering this affliction.

The prevalence of obesity in children is increasing and ranges between 10 and 30 percent of the population, depending on age group and definition of obesity. Statistics from a recent article in the journal *Science* show that obesity among 6 to 11-year-olds has increased by more than 50 percent in the past couple of decades and, what's more, 40 percent of these children will become obese adults. Using the medical definition that one is obese when body weight is 25 to 30 percent greater than that considered standard in actuarial tables, at least 25 percent of Americans are obese. Though there is no consensus on how to prevent childhood obesity, studies have identified certain risk factors and made dietary and behavioral recommendations aimed at reducing the risk.

According to the American Academy of Pediatrics, the major cause of obesity in children is an energy imbalance, where food intake exceeds energy expenditure. Why? is the question. A normal individual's weight does not vary more than 1 to 2 percent over many years. This is because of a delicate physiological balance that is controlled by the brain and is a combination of our perception of hunger and our perception of satiety. It involves blood glucose levels, hormones, and other physical factors. On the other hand, appetite is an emotional factor involving our anticipation of pleasure. It is a learned response to a psychological rather than nutritional state. For obese people, their appetite appears to dominate their brain-controlled hunger and satiety levels.

In modern Western society, this appetite imbalance combined with an abundance of food and an increased reliance on automobiles, labor-saving devices, and passive recreation has led to more and more fat people. While some research has identified a familial predisposition to obesity, it is unclear whether this is due to genetic factors or simply due to learned habits of eating and exercise. Certainly, we inherit the body stature of our parents, but most experts believe that to succumb to this genetic theory of obesity is a fundamental cop-out. Feeding and exercise habits, learned in infancy, are part of the family conditioning that makes the separation of genetic and environmental effects difficult. Stressful life situations, such as school dissatisfaction, parental or peer disapproval, relocation, etc., often contribute to the disruption of normal eating habits. Eating sometimes becomes an adaptive mechanism in the search for happiness, both on the part of the parents and the child. There is also a significant correlation between obesity in adulthood and socioeconomic level. For women, there is a 30 percent incidence among the lower socioeconomic level, 18 percent in the middle level, and only 5 percent in the upper level. This tells us clearly that the problem involves environment, educational level, and beliefs and is not due only to genetics. This is good news because it indicates that obesity is clearly preventable.

Rapid weight gain in infancy has been correlated with adult obesity. Obesity in infancy and childhood can have long-range consequences, for it is associated with an increase in the total number of fat cells as well as the size of fat cells. Obesity in adults usually results only in an increase in the size of fat cells. Thus, it pays to be alert from the start to the possibility of your baby becoming overweight. Once we gain fat cells, we never lose them, and, if we have twice as many fat cells, we will be twice as fat. This doesn't mean that fat babies are doomed to be fat adults, but it does tell us to pay attention to the habits we are establishing from birth.

Obesity Prevention

The American Academy of Pediatrics has made some specific recommendations aimed at preventing obesity. These include:

1. Breast-feed and delay the introduction of solid foods. Many physicians believe that bottle-fed babies who are given solid foods at an early age are actually overfed.

Breast-feeding tends to regulate the amount of milk a baby can get, and overfeeding is much less of a problem.

2. Feed babies only when they are hungry. Do not use food as a pacifier, a reward, or a bribe. When every discomfort is misinterpreted as hunger, your child learns that food is a way of coping with problems. If food is given as an expression of love, your child will turn to food in times of unhappiness or despair. Much adult obesity can be traced to overeating as a coping mechanism in times of stress and depression. Avoid endowing food with emotional ties.

3. Adopt a low-calorie diet. This would include eating plenty of vegetables, fruits, and whole-grain fibers. Obesity is rare in cultures with high-fiber diets. Reduce consumption of fats, which have twice as many calories per gram as proteins and carbohydrates, and limit the amount of sweets and refined carbohydrates in your diet. The disease prevention diet outlined in Chapter 6 is consistent with these recommendations. Remember, this recommendation does not apply to children under the age of two.

4. Establish distinct mealtimes and rules for mealtime behavior. Children need this discipline to learn to eat at specific times, in response to hunger, rather than appetite. Snacking all day long encourages eating to satisfy the appetite.

5. Promote exercise. This may be the single most important step you can take. Studies have shown that obese children are more passive than their slimmer peers. In fact, recent research into the causes of childhood obesity has identified a strong correlation between television watching and obesity. Children who watch a lot of TV get less exercise and tend to eat while they watch. These children also tend to eat the very junk food that is advertised on TV. In addition, these studies recorded a dose effect—that is, the more TV a child watches, the more obese he tends to be.

If your child does become obese, he should be treated early. Chance of successful treatment diminishes as the child grows older. Treated at age 4 to 6, children have been able to lose weight and remain free of weight problems for the rest of their lives. The prognosis is not so optimistic for teenagers and adults. Research now reveals that a life of repeated dieting simply trains the body to become metabolically efficient—the body adapts to functioning on a starvation diet without losing weight. This is why so many people try so hard and so long without success.

Sugars and Sugar Substitutes

While we're talking about obesity, we should straighten out some facts about sugars, sugar substitutes, and highly refined carbohydrates. Sugar, per se, is not a harmful dietary constituent. It is the *overconsumption* of sugar that is harmful. Fifty years ago, per capita sugar consumption in the United States was 25 pounds per year. Now, it is 127 pounds annually! Our children are being brought up as sugar addicts.

This craving or need for large quantities of sugar is not something we are born with. The more sugar we consume, the more we crave. Therefore, the time to start a sugar restriction program is with our babies, before their sugar thresholds are raised. High-sugar diets contribute to weight problems, behavior problems, inability to concentrate, and may lead to maturity-onset diabetes. Here's how sugar effects your body:

Metabolism of Sugar

Blood glucose (blood sugar) is the major energy source for our body. It is the only energy source for our brain and nervous system. When blood glucose levels remain within the normal range, we function efficiently. As they drop below normal, our brain senses the change and we become hungry.

High-sugar foods and highly refined carbohydrates require little digestion and enter the bloodstream quickly in the form of glucose. They can elevate blood glucose levels far above the normal range. This causes a stimulation of the nervous system, which may be expressed, especially in children, as hyperactivity, anxiety, aggressiveness, and an inability to concentrate.

The body reacts to this elevated blood glucose level by producing insulin to metabolize the glucose and lower the blood levels. If the sugar challenge is great, the amount of insulin produced will be great. This often produces a rapid fall in blood glucose to levels below the normal range. Low blood sugar may produce symptoms of irritability, anxiety, fatigue, headache, and clouded thinking. In addition, we become hungry, thus setting the cycle in motion again.

It is easy to see how high-sugar diets can contribute to overeating as well as to serious behavioral and learning problems in children. Unfortunately, they have an even more detrimental effect on weight control. Insulin is the hormone responsible for creating body fat. Each time insulin secretion is stimulated, the excess glucose is stored as body fat. In addition, many experts believe such constant stimulation of insulin production may lead to maturity-onset diabetes. So you see, we have many reasons for wanting to avoid high blood glucose levels, especially in our children.

Natural Sugars

There are a large number of sugars that exist in nature and are employed as commercial sweeteners. Chemically, they are defined either as complex or simple sugars. Your body can utilize only simple sugars and converts the foods you eat into these smaller units. Different foods contain different types and amounts of sugar. For instance, table sugar is a complex sugar that is called sucrose. It is composed of two simple sugars, glucose and fructose. Sucrose is found naturally in cane sugar and in most fruits and vegetables. Honey is also composed of glucose and fructose, but it contains a larger proportion of fructose. Fructose is much sweeter than glucose, hence honey is much sweeter than table sugar. Corn sweetener contains large amounts of fructose and has become a popular ingredient in soft drinks because of its sweetness and lower cost. Lactose is the sugar found in milk, while maltose is a constituent of grains. Table 5.1 lists some of these common sugars, their usual sources, and uses.

Table 5.1.

NATURAL SUGARS

Sugar	Source	Use
sucrose	cane sugar, fruits, vegetables	table sugar, prepared foods
fructose	breakdown product of sucrose, honey, fruits	soft drinks, corn sweetener
glucose (dextrose)	breakdown product of sucrose	I.V. nutrition, commercial sweetener
maltose	grains	alcoholic beverages, commercial sweetener
lactose	milk	component of milk products

Much of the conventional wisdom regarding the different sugars is erroneous. If there are any benefits or risks inherent in eating one form of sugar over another, it will be related to the contaminants present or to the overall nutritive value of the foods eaten. For instance, honey is no more healthful than table sugar. It contains certain bacterial contaminants and traces of bee pollen. Because of this potentially toxic contamination, it should *never* be fed to young babies. Raw or turbinado sugar, long endowed by health-food advocates with beneficial qualities, is actually nothing more than table sugar with natural contaminants such as bacteria, yeast, and molds still present. Brown sugar is actually table sugar with molasses added. Molasses is an intermediate product in the refinement of sugar and contains considerable amounts of vitamins and minerals. Blackstrap molasses is the more nutritious version, but most people don't like its taste.

The important thing to note about the various sugars is their glucose-releasing potential—that is, how effective they are at raising blood glucose and blood insulin levels. Lactose and fructose have little effect on blood glucose levels. Eating milk products, fruit, or foods containing these forms of sugar will not contribute to overly high blood glucose levels. However, fructose does increase the blood concentration of triglycerides (fats). Sucrose has a moderate glucose-elevating potential, but glucose and maltose (both commercial sweeteners) have pronounced effects. Since 80 percent of the sugar in our diet comes in packaged foods, it pays to read labels and avoid products sweetened with glucose and maltose.

A well-balanced diet, as recommended in Chapter 6, will help to prevent the up and down yo-yo effect experienced when glucose is suddenly raised by a sugary snack and subsequently lowered by an increase in blood insulin levels. Generally, highly refined, processed foods cause blood glucose levels to rise sharply. There is no need to avoid sugar as many people do. But, keep your consumption within moderate levels by controlling the intake of soft drinks, sugary snacks, desserts, and commercially prepared foods.

Sugar Substitutes

You may ask that if excess sugar consumption sets off such an undesirable chain of events, why not use sugar substitutes? After all, we are now told that NutraSweet is as natural as bananas and milk! This advertising campaign is misleading. The best one can say about NutraSweet right now is that, unlike saccharin and cyclamates, it does not appear to cause cancer. There are many undesirable health effects to be considered other than cancer.

NutraSweet, or aspartame, as it is called in scientific language, is composed of two amino acids, phenylalanine and aspartic acid. Amino acids, as you recall, are the building blocks of protein and, hence, can be thought of as naturally occurring substances. Remember that your body needs a balanced supply of the different amino acids; nature never packages amino acids alone. Thus, there is a significant difference between aspartame and bananas and milk.

But that's not all. No one really knows what the consequences are of long-term, elevated consumption of these two amino acids, but there are some educated guesses. It is known that phenylalanine is active in brain chemistry. One disorder associated with phenylalanine is phenylketonuria (PKU). This genetic disorder, which affects 1 in 15,000 babies, is characterized by the inability to metabolize phenylalanine. If left untreated, the buildup of phenylalanine in the brain causes mental retardation and seizures. That is why newborn babies are routinely given PKU tests. Aspartame-containing products carry a warning label for sufferers of PKU. But what about the rest of us? It has been estimated that between one and five percent of the population (perhaps as many as ten million people!) unknowingly carry the PKU trait. For them, there may be no safe level of aspartame, for they, too, may have an impaired ability to process phenylalanine. In fact, in anyone with a tendency toward headaches or seizures there may be no safe level of aspartame.

Elevated levels of phenylalanine in normal people can interfere with the delicate chemistry of the brain, affecting our thinking, behavior, and moods. Side effects can include headaches, migraines, dizziness, depression, panic attacks, seizures, insomnia, rashes, mood swings, high blood pressure, and behavior and learning problems. Ironically, aspartame is consumed by diet-conscious people in an effort to control weight. Yet, substantial evidence indicates that it actually upsets our brain's appetite control center, causing us to overeat. This is crucially important, for it is an imbalance in our appetite control center that causes obesity.

Normally, how much aspartame is safe? That depends on a number of individual factors and also on what you eat along with it. If you drink your diet soda with a high carbohydrate snack (like pretzels), the carbohydrates will stimulate the production of insulin. Insulin selectively lowers the levels of other competitive amino acids entering the brain. This enables more phenylalanine to enter the brain. If, however, you consume aspartame with a protein snack, the other amino acids will probably have a moderating effect, and less phenylalanine will enter the brain.

As mentioned earlier, children are far more sensitive to chemicals in our food supply. Unborn babies, children, and teenagers are particularly susceptible to the effects of aspartame, for their brains are undergoing rapid development. An imbalance in brain chemistry at these ages can have far-reaching effects. Consumption of aspartame by pregnant women may increase the risk of neurological birth defects such as mild mental retardation. Naturally, this risk extends throughout the lactating period. Many neurobiologists believe there are no safe levels of consumption for pregnant and lactating women and for children under the age of four.

Why did the FDA approve aspartame if it has so many drawbacks? To understand this question, you must understand the system under which the FDA operates. It is not the responsibility of the FDA to prove that an additive is harmful. It is the responsibility of the manufacturer to prove, by laboratory and animal testing, that it is "reasonably safe." The Delaney Clause of the Food, Drug, and Cosmetic Act requires manufacturers to prove that the proposed additive *does not cause cancer*. It does not require them to investigate other health hazards. You should keep this in mind when evaluating the risks inherent in all food additives.

Neurobiologists from the Massachusetts Institute of Technology and other leading medical research institutions have recommended against the approval of aspartame by the FDA. Because of the considerable doubts raised, the FDA first limited aspartame use to dry foods and set a maximum safety level. This safety level was set using standard tests; it was not a measure of specific safety to the brain. Now with approval extended to soft drinks and many other products such as vitamins and ice cream, it may be impossible to monitor exposure levels to the general population. In addition, you can't even monitor your own consumption because manufacturers are not required to disclose the amount of aspartame in their products. Over one hundred million people are now involved in a grand experiment that will eventually answer the question "How safe is aspartame?"

For adults, the answer to this question will probably be that moderate consumption of aspartame poses no health problem. But then, neither does moderate consumption of sugar, which is certainly far safer. For children and pregnant and lactating women, the question is far more complex. How are we to measure slight mental impairment? How will we know if a child has failed to reach his full potential? Can we trace subtle behavior or learning problems to this chemical?

To avoid consumption of aspartame by your children, you will have to be on guard. The list of aspartame fortified products grows daily. An aggressive advertising campaign

directed toward consumers and intended to create cus-
tomer loyalty to aspartame has now extended its use to a
variety of children's products such as gelatin desserts, fruit
drinks, puddings, ice cream, cereals, even orange juice,
yogurt, and children's vitamins! Read labels carefully.

Hypertension

Hypertension, or chronic high blood pressure, is the
most common medical problem in the United States today,
affecting 1 in 5 adults. It is one of the most powerful risk
factors in the development of coronary artery disease and
stroke; it also contributes to diseases of the kidneys and
eyes. Because hypertension usually takes twenty to forty
years to develop, it too should be considered a pediatric
problem. Though onset is generally after age 30, underlying
physiological changes begin occurring early in life. Children of hypertensive parents often begin to exhibit elevated
blood pressures at surprisingly young ages—sometimes in
their teens.

Should we be so overly concerned? After all, everyone
knows that this disease can be treated. This is correct, and
hypertension, though incurable, can be controlled with
drugs. However, reliable control of blood pressure through
drugs is often difficult to achieve and may be accompanied
by severe side effects. In addition, we must remember that
drugs are foreign substances and may present unforeseen
risks. With some understanding of this disease and the
factors in our diets that contribute to high blood pressure,
we can raise our children in a way that will reduce their risk
of developing high blood pressure and its consequences,
coronary heart disease and stroke.

How do we get high blood pressure? Scientists aren't
completely sure. The system that regulates our blood pres-

sure is very complex and influenced by many different factors, some of them dietary, some of them genetic, and some of them emotional. The three most important risk factors are heredity, salt intake, and obesity, though recent studies suggest strongly that other nutritional factors such as calcium intake, may have profound effects. It appears that hypertension may develop over time, when we ingest more sodium (primarily as salt) than our kidneys are capable of excreting. The extra sodium remaining in our tissues causes our body to retain more water, thus expanding our blood volume. This creates more pressure in our circulatory system, just as blowing more air into a balloon creates more pressure on the walls of the balloon. It also makes our heart work harder. Many hormonal and cellular effects occur as our bodies try to compensate for this stressful condition.

You can see why a lifelong diet that is high in salt can lead to high blood pressure. This is particularly true of the 10 percent of the population who are born "salt-sensitive." For these people, a genetically impaired kidney with reduced sodium excretion capacity puts them at a higher than normal risk. This is why a family history of high blood pressure is important in the development of this disease.

Obesity is another significant risk factor. In fact, obesity in young adulthood has been shown to be a predictor of hypertension. Excessive eating appears to stimulate the overproduction of insulin, which then causes your body to retain more sodium. An ideal weight, especially in the period of young adulthood, may be an important preventive measure to avoid subsequent development of hypertension. Your child's weight as he approaches adulthood will depend on how well you have taught him the basics of nutrition and disease prevention.

Many people think that blood pressure increases with age; the older you get, the higher your blood pressure. This is only true in populations whose weight also increases with age. Blood pressure increases with weight, not with age.

Sodium is not the only nutritional factor that has been correlated with hypertension. Dietary calcium is the single best nutritional predictor of blood pressure. Although the exact role that calcium plays in hypertension is not known, it has been suggested that its function in maintaining water balance and in muscle cell and arterial functioning are important aspects of its mode of action. Studies show that people on high-calcium diets have a lower incidence of hypertension. It may not be surprising to learn that in the United States, where at least 20 percent of the population suffers from hypertension, calcium deficiency is the number one nutritional deficiency. An estimated 50 to 70 percent of the population fails to get the recommended daily supply of calcium. In fact, half of the children in the United States do not get sufficient calcium to support the needs of their growing bones. Such a deficiency early in life may contribute to the development of high blood pressure.

The best way to obtain calcium is to eat a diet rich in calcium-containing foods such as milk, milk products, and green leafy vegetables. If your consumption of milk products is low, you may need to take a calcium supplement to meet the RDA requirements (see Appendix A). If you choose a calcium supplement, you should be aware that doses above the RDA may be associated with kidney stones.

Potassium is another dietary component whose deficiency causes an increased risk for hypertension. Like calcium, potassium is involved in muscle cell function and fluid volume factors and is thus important to cardiovascular regulation. Our bodies have a relatively large requirement for potassium, but fortunately, this nutrient is ubiquitous, found especially in fresh fruits, vegetables, and dairy products. Those people at risk for consuming less than the RDA will probably be eating fewer fresh foods and more prepared foods.

According to a 1984 report published in *Science*, deficiencies in vitamins A and C may also be associated with an increased risk of hypertension. Little is known about the role of these two vitamins in the regulation of blood pressure, but it is known that vitamin A is closely associated with calcium and vitamin C with potassium. Considering that neither vitamin is harmful at RDA intakes, it would be best to make sure you get your daily quota.

Dietary fats, the real villains in our food supply, have also been linked to high blood pressure. A 1984 hypertension workshop conducted by the National Institutes of Health reported that blood pressure is raised with a high-fat diet rich in saturated fat. Blood pressure can be significantly reduced with a low-fat diet, high in polyunsaturated fats. High-fiber diets have also been shown to reduce blood pressure, though it is not known whether this is due to the inherently lower fat intake or the higher fiber content. What is emerging as a consistent pattern for the promotion of many different disease states is a diet high in fats, low in fiber, and deficient in certain vitamins and minerals.

Osteoporosis

Osteoporosis is a disease of bone degeneration in which bone mineral is lost, causing the bones to become brittle and to break easily. It is generally a disease of aging, especially prevalent in postmenopausal women. It can, however, occur in children if there is a dietary deficiency. This is common in premature infants who can not be fed enough calcium and phosphorous to support their relatively high growth rates and is also seen in children if they have a metabolic problem which prevents full utilization of the nutrients they consume.

The best protection against osteoporosis is an ample supply of calcium during the growing years. Recent evidence suggests that calcium supplementation in middle age may have no effect in retarding the progression of osteoporosis in old age. To spare your daughter from this risk, be sure that she receives the RDA for dietary calcium through her teenage years. Since calcium deficiency has been identified as affecting 50 percent of school-age children in this country, it makes sense to pay attention to the calcium in your child's diet.

Nutrition and Dental Caries

Your child's dental health is another aspect of his overall health that is influenced by what he eats. One of the most significant public health discoveries is the relationship between dietary fluoride and a reduction in dental caries. A large number of studies have demonstrated this relationship and produced specific recommendations for fluoridation of public drinking water at safe and effective levels. Since the 1950s, fluoride supplementation, either through drinking water or vitamin preparations, has resulted in a 50 to 60 percent reduction in tooth decay. If your water supply is not fluoridated, your physician can prescribe a fluoride-vitamin combination to protect your child's developing teeth. While these preparations are less desirable than the constant dose received in drinking water, they are still an acceptable alternative.

But since some kids do still get cavities, here are some things you should do to reduce the likelihood of your child spending a lot of time in the dentist's chair.

1. Limit dietary sugar. Sugar is an essential ingredient for the initiation of tooth decay, for it is the food on which tooth-destroying bacteria thrive. Sucrose (table sugar) is the most cariogenic of sugars; but all sugars contribute to this bacterial process.

2. Encourage frequent brushing. Bacteria and sugar residues are removed and reduced with regular brushing.

3. Discourage frequent snacking, especially sugary snacks. When bacterial plaque comes into contact with sugar, an enamel-dissolving acid is produced for at least 20 minutes. The more frequent snacking, the more challenge to the teeth.

4. Eat sugary foods at mealtimes along with foods that are rich in proteins and fats. Both proteins and fats have the ability to buffer this salivary acid and reduce its cariogenic qualities.

5. Avoid sticky sweet snacks, such as honey, toffee, and dried fruits. Their consistencies increase their contact time and prolong their acid-producing potential.

Summary

Obesity

It has been estimated that 25 percent of American children are obese, and the problem is growing. Prevention may hold the only hope for this disease, which historically has been extremely difficult to treat successfully. Alertness on the part of parents to the causes of childhood obesity can help in prevention. Here are the key points to remember:

1. Breast-feed and delay the introduction of solid foods.

2. Feed your baby only when he is hungry. Do not use food to bribe or reward your child.

3. Provide your family with a well-balanced, low-calorie diet that includes plenty of fresh fruits, vegetables, and fiber. This will set the stage and provide a healthy diet for your two-year-old when he is ready.

4. Establish firm mealtime rules.

5. Promote physical exercise. Discourage TV watching and mindless snacking.

6. Keep your consumption of sweets in perspective.

Hypertension

High blood pressure affects 20 percent of adult Americans and is the leading risk factor in heart disease, stroke, and atherosclerosis. Though onset is usually after age 30, the disease is silently working early in life. Here are important facts to remember in preventing hypertension:

1. Keep your salt consumption down. Once you get used to unsalted foods you will be surprised at the delicate flavors you were hiding. For your baby, start him on a diet that contains no added salt, and he'll always enjoy the natural good taste of foods. Remember that most prepared foods contain large amounts of salt.

2. Maintain an ideal body weight.

3. Be sure to get your RDA of calcium each day.

4. To assure yourself of adequate potassium intake, be sure to eat plenty of fresh fruits, vegetables, and dairy products.

5. Adults and children over 2 should eat a low-fat diet that substitutes polyunsaturated fats for saturated fats.

6. Adults and children over 2 should add fiber to their diets.

Osteoporosis

Resistance to osteroporosis in later life is dependent on healthy bone formation during the growing years. Be sure that your children receive adequate calcium while their bones are developing.

Dental Caries

Tooth decay has almost become a thing of the past. Here are the things to do to assure your children of good oral health:

1. Be sure your children receive adequate fluoride protection, either through fluoridated public drinking water or physician-prescribed supplements.

2. Limit the amount of sugar in your children's diets and discourage between-meal snacking.

3. Provide sugary foods in moderation at mealtimes along with foods balanced in protein and fat content.

4. Encourage frequent brushing.

CHAPTER 5: REFERENCES

1. American Academy of Pediatrics. *Pediatric Nutrition Handbook*. Elk Grove Village, IL, 1985.

2. American Academy of Allergy and Immunology Committee on Adverse Reactions to Foods. *Adverse Reactions to Foods*. National Institutes of Health Publication No. 84-2442, 1984.

3. *NIH Workshop on Nutrition and Hypertension: Proceedings from a Symposium*. New York: Biomedical Information Corporation, 1984.

4. Kolata, Gina. "Dietary Dogma Disproved," *Science* 1983. 220:487–488.

5. McCarron, D. et al. "Blood Pressure and Nutrient Intake in the United States," *Science* 1984. 224:1392–1398.

6. Sidney Blumenthal, M.D., Ed. *Hypertension: Prevention, Diet, and Treatment in Infancy and Childhood*. Proceedings from a symposium, Bethesda, MD, May 25, 1983.

7. Wurtman, R. "Neurochemical changes following high-dose aspartame with dietary carbohydrates," *N Eng J Med* 1983. 309:429–430.

8. Wurtman, R. "Possible Relationship Between Aspartame (Nutra-Sweet) Consumption, Seizures, and Other CNS Abnormalities." Introductory comments presented to the FDA, April 21, 1986.

Section Two

FEEDING GUIDELINES

CHAPTER 6

Nutritional Guidelines for the Whole Family

Now that we've seen how the excesses and deficiencies in the average American diet contribute to the development of the major chronic diseases, it's time to put this information to work for your baby and your family. We have reviewed the dietary factors influencing the development of many different disease states, and again and again the same foods emerge as the culprits. It is the rich American diet, heavy in fats, light in fiber, that causes high rates of cancer, heart disease, atherosclerosis, hypertension, and obesity. Combine this diet with low exercise, and any child is on the path toward at least one of the chronic diseases.

We can no longer ignore the warnings of the medical profession. While these diseases generally emerge in middle to later life, there is compelling evidence that they begin their destructive processes in childhood. It's never too late to begin a disease-prevention diet, but obviously the sooner you start, the better. An infant's body has not yet been assaulted by harmful substances, his tissues and organs are new and are in perfect health. He also has not yet formed opinions and food preferences and is free of harmful eating habits. If you begin with an informed approach, providing the right nutrients and avoiding the hazardous ones, you can help your child achieve a state of health that he can enjoy throughout life.

The complexity of today's world presents us with unique challenges, but it has also begun to provide us with the knowledge necessary to keep the human body healthy for a lifetime. Just as advances in nutrition over the years have produced taller generations, discoveries linking foods and disease will help our children live longer, healthier lives. These goals can be realized if the whole family adopts a disease-prevention diet; children learn from the examples set by their parents.

This chapter gives you practical help in implementing an all-around disease-prevention diet for the whole family. It summarizes the major points presented in Chapters 1 through 5 and gives you examples of foods to avoid and foods to add to your diet. Best of all, the facts are simple and easy to remember. You will not need to consult this book every time you plan a meal.

Infants have specialized needs and can not be started on an adult disease-prevention diet before the age of 2. To do so would compromise their growth and development and increase their risk of disease. Specific and detailed guidelines are given in Chapters 8 through 10 for babies up to the age of 2. Read each one as your baby progresses to each new stage. After age 2, your baby can begin to eat the same diet as the rest of the family.

Eating to Avoid Chronic Diseases

It's really remarkable how simple it all is and how much sense it makes. There are only a few things you need to keep in mind.

1. *Eat a wide variety of foods.*

* By eating foods from the four basic food groups each day, you are assured of providing your family with a balanced diet that provides all the essential nutrients.

* By varying the foods you serve every day, you will minimize the risk of developing food allergies.

* And in today's world, if we make it a habit to eat many different foods, we protect ourselves from excessive exposure to any one contaminant.

2. *Reduce your consumption of dietary components implicated in disease.*

* Top on this list are total fats, saturated fats, and cholesterol. It may be difficult to give up your whipped cream and fried chicken, but this is probably the single most important step to take in reducing the risk of cancer, heart disease, atherosclerosis, and obesity.

* Reduce your consumption of other foods suspected of causing cancer (see Chapter 3 for specifics) and hazardous food additives (see Appendix E).

* Avoid excess consumption of sugars and highly refined, processed, and packaged foods. They provide a lot of calories, but few basic materials for building and maintaining healthy bodies. They contribute to obesity and overall poor health.

* Avoid too much sodium, one of the prime risk factors in the development of high blood pressure.

3. *Add protective factors to your diet.*

* Eat plenty of fresh fruits and vegetables, for they supply many vitamins, minerals, and other protective factors and an abundance of fiber, all of which fight cancer and help reduce blood cholesterol levels. Being generally low in calories, they also help to prevent obesity.

* Add fiber to your diet. Vegetables, fruits and whole-grain breads and cereals provide bulky indigestible food components that speed the elimination of food wastes and protect the digestive system from disease.

* Serve more fish meals, especially the oily fish that are high in Omega 3 oils.

* Substitute polyunsaturated fats for saturated ones wherever prudent.

* Be sure to get your RDA of calcium each day to avoid hypertension and osteoporosis.

4. *Take an age-appropriate multivitamin and mineral supplement each day.*

It insures adequate intake of important nutrients and protective factors.

As you put these recommendations to work for your family, it is important to adopt a balanced perspective. Eliminating all dietary risk factors from your life is not only impossible, it is also inadvisable. Many important foods contain components that have been implicated in disease. The best approach is to weigh the benefits with the risks. Eliminate those high-risk foods that have little nutritional value and try to limit your consumption of other foods that you now know contribute to disease. This is relatively easy to do and will leave you more room to add foods with protective factors to boost your self-defense system. Adding these protective factors by way of some delicious and nutritious food choices puts you on a path to better overall health and carries no additional risk. Here are some practical tips to get you started.

Reducing the Fat Content of Your Meals

Your greatest challenge will be to reduce the fat content of your meals. It won't be easy, and there will be some resistance. After all, everyone loves whipped cream! But if you approach it creatively, you will be surprised at how easy the conversion will be. And you needn't think of it as total denial. People who eat a low-fat diet are not compromised when at Thanksgiving they top off their pumpkin pie with a little whipped cream.

First you must learn to recognize dietary fat. It's easy to see the fat trimming a piece of steak or marbling a ham. But even after you've discarded this visible fat, meats still contain a substantial amount of fat hidden within their fibers. But there are foods you may not think are high in fat yet are. For instance, tastewise, there's very little difference between low-fat yogurt and whole-milk yogurt; yet the fat content will be substantially different.

And as we have already learned, not all fats are created equal. How harmful a food is as a dietary component will depend on the type of fat as well as the total fat content. So, let's look at what steps we can take to improve our menus.

1. *Keep in mind the foods that are high in total fat, saturated fat, or cholesterol.* These are some of the most important foods to avoid or serve less often. Table 6.1 includes some of them.

2. *Select lean meats and trim all visible fat before cooking.* Invest in a good pair of kitchen scissors. It will make the trimming much easier. Generally, prime cuts of meat have more hidden fat than the less expensive grades. The opposite is true with ground meats; the less expensive they are, the higher the fat content.

Reduce servings of red meats to less than five times per week, and reduce the size of individual servings.

3. *Eat more poultry and fish.* Be sure to remove all visible fat from poultry, and, whenever possible, remove the skin before cooking. Fifty percent of the fat on a chicken is in the skin. To prevent skinned chicken pieces from drying during baking, coat with breadcrumbs or wrap in foil.

Table 6.1.

FOODS HIGH IN TOTAL FAT, SATURATED FAT, OR CHOLESTEROL

fried foods	fast foods
whole milk	rich desserts
whipped cream	nondairy toppings
sour cream	cheddar cheese
American cheese	jack cheese
Swiss cheese	Brie
Camembert	bleu cheese
cream cheese	butter
cream	nondairy creamers
ice cream	red meats
bacon	sausages
luncheon meats	hot dogs
organ meats	pie crust
nuts	frostings
chocolate	potato chips
avocados	olives
peanut butter	

4. *Eliminate fried foods from your menus.* Oven-broil, bake, roast, microwave, or steam instead. Try sautéing in broth or even a little water instead of in oil or butter. Use pans with no-stick surfaces that reduce or eliminate the need for fat.

If your family is really resistant to giving up fried chicken, try coating skinned chicken pieces with crushed crackers, cereal, or other crispy coating and bake in the oven.

5. *Substitute low-fat dairy products for whole-milk products.*

* Serve skim milk or low-fat milk to everyone over 2 years old.

* Switch from ice cream to ice milk or sherbet.
* Be sure to buy low-fat yogurt.
* Use low-fat yogurt instead of sour cream for toppings, dips, salad dressings, recipes. Try it as a frosting on cake.

*Select low-fat cheeses, such as partially skim milk mozzarella, cottage, farmer, ricotta, or "light" processed American cheese. Avoid the rich cheeses, such as Brie, Camembert, cream cheese, and others made from full fat milk.

* Use more buttermilk. Contrary to its name, buttermilk contains no fat and enhances the flavor of many recipes. Try it in salad dressings, cakes, biscuits, and pancakes.

6. *Do not eat at fast-food restaurants.* Look for family restaurants that give you the choice of a broad menu with salad bars, basic sandwiches, fish, chicken, broiled and baked entrees, etc.

Adding Protective Factors to Your Menus

Adding foods containing protective factors to our diets will reduce the challenge to our immune systems and help our bodies counteract different disease processes. Once you learn to recognize the foods that contain these protective factors, it's an easy matter to get your family to eat them. Luckily, as you will see, many foods are nutritionally dense—that is, they contain high levels of several nutrients that have protective qualities. This makes your job a lot easier and the list of foods to remember a lot smaller.

Table 6.2 presents a number of foods that are high in specific nutrients identified as beneficial in disease prevention.

Table 6.2.

FOODS RICH IN PROTECTIVE FACTORS

Cruciferous Vegetables

broccoli	cabbage
Brussels sprouts	cauliflower
rutabagas	turnips

Foods high in vitamin A and beta-carotene
(Dark yellow, orange, and green)

carrots	apricots
sweet potato	peaches
broccoli	nectarines
tomatoes	cantaloup
winter squash	watermelon
spinach	cherries
kale	Swiss chard
endive	pumpkin
mustard greens	asparagus
beet greens	collards

Foods high in vitamin C

orange	broccoli
grapefruit	Brussels sprouts
lemon	cauliflower
lime	collards
cantaloup	kale
cranberries	mustard greens
papaya	green peppers
strawberries	spinach
pineapples	citrus juices

Foods high in fiber

fruits	vegetables
bran	granola
wheat germ	whole wheat
brown rice	oatmeal
barley	rye

seeds   nuts
kidney beans   lima beans
pinto beans   navy beans
white beans   chick peas
blackberries   dried prunes

Fish high in Omega 3 oils

salmon   herring
swordfish   tuna
snapper   mackerel
sardines   trout
pompano   lake whitefish

Polyunsaturated oils

safflower   sunflower
corn   wheat germ
soybean

Foods high in calcium

milk   cheese
yogurt   buttermilk
custards   puddings
ice milk   clams
fish   oysters
sardines   shrimp
almonds   beet greens
broccoli   bok choy cabbage
collards   kale
mustard greens   spinach
rhubarb   blackstrap molasses

Foods high in potassium

fruits   vegetables
milk   nuts
bran   lentils
beef   chicken
clams   fish
molasses

Adding Fiber to Your Diet

One of the easiest and most enjoyable ways to add fiber to your diet is to eat more fresh fruits and vegetables. Push fresh fruits, kids love them anyway. But go easy on fruit juices. While they do contain vitamins, they usually have little if any fiber. Vegetables may be a little more difficult for children to accept. Pick up a creative vegetable cookbook (see the Suggested Reading list in Appendix F) to give you some ideas. Be careful not to overcook your vegetables. It destroys vitamins, reduces the value of the fiber, and robs them of good taste.

Try adding fiber to your desserts and baked goods. Chapter 12 will give you some ideas on how to do this. Basically, just take your favorite recipes and use half white flour and half whole wheat flour. Or try substituting 1/4 to 1/2 cup of wheat germ for an equivalent amount of flour in your cookie recipes. You'll be surprised at the nice, nutty flavor that results. You can also add oatmeal, bran, or granola cereal to cookie recipes.

Buy only whole-grain breads. Kids may put up a fuss at first, but they will adjust.

Choose whole-grain, bran, granola, or oatmeal cereals, hot or cold, for breakfast, instead of a piece of white toast or a sugary donut.

Serve dried beans. Kidney, navy, pinto, white beans, lentils and chick peas, all contain substantial amounts of beneficial fiber, as do lima beans.

Use brown rice instead of overly processed white rice. Try some new and interesting grains, like barley or bulghur.

Avoiding Highly Allergenic Foods

You can develop an allergy to any food, but it is the foods you eat most often that are likely to cause problems.

That's why eating moderate quantities of a wide variety of different foods will help protect you from food allergies. In addition, some foods are implicated more often than others in the development of allergies. Learn to recognize the highly allergenic foods listed in Tables 6.3 and 6.4 so that your family may eat them with caution.

Table 6.3.

FOODS MOST LIKELY TO CAUSE ALLERGIES

milk and milk products	pork
egg white	fish
wheat	shellfish
corn	nuts (especially peanuts)
peas	peanut butter
citrus fruits	tomatoes
yeast	sugar
berries	food colorings
chocolate	cola drinks
cinnamon	mustard

Table 6.4.

FOODS THAT MAY CAUSE ALLERGIES

beef	apples
chicken	bananas
coffee	cherries
potatoes	prunes
mushrooms	plums
onions	melons
garlic	lettuce
spices	celery
soybeans	

Health Factors Other Than Diet

There are considerations other than dietary ones that contribute to your health. Exercise ranks high among the life-style factors that influence the development of disease. It is well known that unused muscles atrophy. A body which is not regularly called upon to exert energy will lose some of its ability to respond when called upon. Exercise improves the ability of all the body systems to meet challenges. An active life is one of your family's best insurance policies.

Maintaining ideal body weight is yet another essential element in disease prevention. As we have seen, obesity increases the risk of developing all of the chronic diseases and carries with it some serious emotional problems. Excess weight makes it more difficult for your body to perform its routine functions. All organs and systems are stressed. Fortunately, a disease-prevention diet, started early enough, will help avert this problem.

Your overall mental health, your attitude toward life and your personality traits are other important components of health. Research is just now beginning to elucidate the role of the nervous system in controlling the various immune functions. Depression, anxiety, and stress can significantly impede the ability of your immune system to react properly to challenges.

Cigarette smoking is, of course, a primary contributor to many diseases, for it suppresses your immune system's capabilities. This will probably not be a problem for your children if you educate them about the dangers of smoking. In fact, for today's youth, peer pressure often has the positive effect of turning them away from cigarette smoking. For yourself, if you're still smoking, this should be the area in which to begin your disease prevention program. Your child will learn from your example.

Environmental factors can also add to your disease

risk. For instance, if you live in an area of dense chemical pollution or contamination, you will be at increased risk for developing cancer. If your occupation exposes you to biological hazards, that, too, will contribute to the risk. If it is not possible to remove these dangers from your life, adding dietary protective factors can help mitigate the deleterious effects of such environmental components.

Heredity is the final primary factor determining your overall state of health. It may appear that you have little control over your genetic destiny, but this is not wholly accurate. Even if you are born with a predisposition to a particular disease, you can significantly influence the final outcome. The eventual development of most of the major diseases is dependent on a complex interplay of diet and all the foregoing factors. By actively working with the factors that are under your control, you can greatly minimize the role of your genes.

Summary

Use the suggestions and tables in this chapter to help you establish a disease-prevention diet for your whole family. Remember to eat a wide variety of simple, wholesome foods, reduce your consumption of high-risk foods, add protective factors to your diet—and for insurance, take an age-appropriate multivitamin and mineral supplement each day.

CHAPTER 7

Diet of the Nursing Mother

If you are serious about a disease-prevention program for your baby, you will choose to breast-feed unless you are adopting or have health problems that prevent nursing. Human milk has health benefits that go far beyond its nutritional value; it contains immune factors, and it is nature's way of conferring immunity on babies. Since babies are born with immature immune systems, they need help to win against viral and bacterial infections. Breast-feeding also helps the new mother deal with her body's instinct to produce milk and aids in the subsequent emotional bonding that occurs between mother and child. Chapter 8 will discuss in detail the enormous health advantages of breast milk for your baby. This chapter provides the information necessary for you to protect the quality of your milk supply so that it will truly be the optimal food for the growth and health of your baby.

Human milk is a complex mixture of nutrients and immunologic factors. If you are in optimal health and your immune system is operating at its best, you can expect the quality of your milk to be high. However, just about everything you eat and are exposed to can get into your milk supply, so special awareness is necessary to protect your baby from environmental pollutants, chemicals, drugs, and food allergens. Because breast-feeding is a natural process, we tend to forget that human milk is also subject to contamination in today's world.

It is reassuring to know that there are no foods that are either especially beneficial or harmful during lactation, and furthermore, that the nutritional composition of human milk is largely beyond our control. Even the milk from poorly nourished mothers, though reduced in quantity, is surprisingly high in nutritive value. This is, of course, at the expense of maternal nutrient stores. To prevent bone demineralization or other physiological deficiencies, you need to be aware of your increased nutritional needs during lactation. While the protein and caloric content of breast milk is unaffected by maternal diet, the vitamin and fat composition of your milk is determined by the foods you eat, so you will want to pay attention to your requirements for these nutrients to protect your baby from any deficiency.

Before you begin breast-feeding, it is best to read all the information you can find to support you in this endeavor. Because this is so important to the health of your infant, you will want to do everything possible to assure your success. One of the biggest problems in breast-feeding is the failure to establish and maintain lactation. This is most often due to poor maternal attitude, lack of information, lack of family support, or fear of failure. These problems can be overcome with education, a good support structure, and a winning attitude. It is rare to encounter a healthy woman who is physically unable to breast-feed. Remember, you have nature on your side.

For additional resources consult Appendix F, Suggested Reading and contact your local chapter of the La Leche League International. They can provide you with books, pamphlets, and informational guides to answer any questions you might have; but, more importantly, they have women in your community who have breast-fed and who are ready to help you on a personal level. They will help you find a way to fit breast-feeding into your life.

If you still have doubts as to whether or not you want to breast-feed, perhaps you should consider the benefits *you* will derive from it. After spending the last three months of pregnancy with your body contour pretty much out of control, you're probably anxious to return to your normal weight and shape. Breast-feeding is nature's way of helping you attain these goals. First, as your infant nurses, the suckling stimulates the production of the hormone oxytocin, which causes uterine contractions. These contractions help control blood loss and speed the return of your uterus to its prepregnant state. Then as lactation proceeds, your body begins to burn off the 5 or 10 pounds of fat that it purposely stored during pregnancy to help you meet the extra energy requirements of lactation. If you do not breast-feed, you will have to take off that extra weight without any help. For many women, the lifelong battle with the waistline begins after pregnancies that are not followed by lactation.

If you would like to breast-feed but must return to work, don't automatically feel you have to discontinue breast-feeding. Many women have successfully handled both commitments. In fact, breast-feeding can help you maintain a close relationship with your infant and combat any guilt feelings you may develop by having to leave your baby so soon. You can be comforted in the fact that you are still able to share with him the health of your body. Besides, breast-feeding is so much easier than formula feeding; no need for sterilizing bottles and other paraphernalia, no time wasted in preparing, heating, or shopping and no worry about running out of supplies. It's practically hassle-free. And remember, your baby will have fewer health problems, which means, in the long run, that you will miss less work.

To breast-feed while working, you will need to be creative in structuring your day. You may be able to make arrangements to stop by your sitter's during your lunch hour (a pleasurable break in your day!). Or you could give your baby a bottle of expressed breast milk or formula for the missed meal. To assure your infant of the immunological protection of breast milk when he needs it most, you might consider expressing your milk until he is two to three months old and substituting formula thereafter. Some adjustments will be necessary for both you and your baby, so it's best to begin the new routine before you start work. Your breasts will adapt remarkably to just about any schedule if you give them a little time, and your baby will learn to drink from both bottle and breast in spite of the resistance you may encounter initially. It is important to remember that through these efforts you are insuring your baby of the best possible health and nutrition.

Nutritional Requirements of Lactation

Lactation places even greater demands on your body than pregnancy. If you do not meet these increased needs, the quality and quantity of your milk could suffer, and your own health might be compromised. An optimal diet during lactation will provide more of each nutrient in a balanced way, and significantly, it will provide more energy and more protein than your regular diet. Producing milk for your baby requires an additional 500 to 800 calories per day. Nature, in its wisdom, has deliberately stored some body fat to help you meet this huge increase in caloric need. However, you will still need to increase your caloric intake by about 25 percent, or 500 calories per day for the first three months. Thereafter, you will need to consume about 800 extra calories per day to support your baby. These recommendations allow for the gradual loss of those extra pounds stored during pregnancy. No matter how anxious you are to return to a trim body, this is definitely not the time to go on a diet. Even a moderate reduction in your caloric intake can compromise your ability to produce milk, especially in the early weeks.

In addition to extra calories, you will need to consume 65 grams of protein, or nearly 50 percent more protein than normally required. This may seem like a lot, but keep in mind that most Americans consume about 90 grams of protein daily, or twice the protein they actually need. Chances are a modest increase in your protein intake will more than compensate for the demands of lactation.

Though low-fat diets are recommended for disease prevention, it is best not to be too restrictive of your fat intake during lactation. The fat content of your milk is affected by your diet. Human milk has a high fat content (4.5 percent), and it's supposed to. Babies need those extra calories to support their enormous growth, and you need the extra calories of a higher fat diet to support your milk production. This is not a carte blanche to go overboard on whipped cream or fried foods, just a reminder to include healthful sources of fat in your diet.

Also, don't forget to increase your consumption of fluids. You won't make enough milk if you don't drink enough water. You should now be consuming about 2 to 3 quarts of liquids each day. Normal intake is about 2 quarts.

The vitamin content of your milk supply is most influenced by your diet. Now is the time to eat more citrus fruits, fresh vegetables, meats and vegetable oils to assure yourself of a balanced supply of vitamins and minerals. In addition, to guard against deficiency, your physician will most likely prescribe a vitamin and mineral supplement that has been specially formulated for lactation. Check the Appendix A for the Recommended Daily Allowances of each of the vitamins during lactation. The appropriate formulation will not be available without a prescription since the maximum amount of folacin available over the counter is 400 micrograms (µg), and 500 µg is the RDA for lactating women. Folacin is extremely important for proper growth and neurological development.

The mineral content of breast milk is not generally responsive to maternal diet. This means that if you do not consume sufficient quantities to support your milk production, your body will take these nutrients from your own body stores. Calcium is perhaps the most important mineral because its concentration in milk is very high, and its requirement during lactation increases by 50 percent over normal. If you do not include enough sources of calcium in your diet, your baby will not suffer; you will suffer. Calcium will be mobilized from your bones in a process which is suspected to contribute to the development of osteoporosis. For this reason, it is recommended that you increase your consumption of milk products during lactation in addition to taking calcium supplements.

Iron is another mineral you should pay special attention to during lactation. Your iron stores are taxed by both pregnancy and childbirth. Recovering from this induced state of iron-deficiency anemia is long and slow. You should take iron supplements until your physician assures you that your iron levels have returned to normal.

As a general rule, your body's requirement for vitamins and nutrients increases during lactation by 50 to 100 percent over normal. The prescription supplement will take care of some of this, but don't neglect your overall nutrition lest you compromise your own health.

Allergens in Breast Milk

Breast-feeding is the single most important step you can take to prevent the development of allergic disease in your infant. As you have read in Chapter 2, many infant allergies are caused by foods. Since breast milk is the only food known to be nonallergenic to babies, you might think that breast-feeding would guarantee that your baby will not develop an allergy. Unfortunately, this is not the full story. Food allergens from the maternal diet commonly enter breast milk and can cause problems for infants. Awareness of this fact, coupled with a corrective plan of action, can protect your baby.

While the risk of developing allergies in general is something we inherit from our parents, the risk of a breast-fed baby developing an allergy from breast milk does not appear to be related to a family predisposition. It does, however, appear to be related to certain aspects of the mother's immune system. IgA antibodies, one class of immune components present in breast milk, appear to have the ability to remove food allergens from breast milk and prevent them from being passed on to the infant. Studies have demonstrated an association between infant allergic symptoms and a lowered IgA antibody concentration in their mother's milk. At present, there is no practical way to identify women who may have insufficient quantities of IgA antibodies in their breast milk. The best you can do is to maintain good immune health through an optimal diet and exercise, and pay attention to any symptoms of allergic reaction your infant develops.

There are a few things that you can do to minimize the risk of food allergens being passed along to your infant. One thing is to reduce the level of potential immune challenge by being careful not to eat highly allergenic foods. Any of the foods listed in the charts of allergenic foods in Chapter 6 may cause a reaction, but Table 7.1 lists the problem foods that are most likely to pass into breast milk. With the exception of milk and milk products, it is fairly easy to avoid these foods or at least limit your consumption of them.

Table 7.1.

HIGHLY ALLERGENIC FOODS THAT MAY PASS INTO BREAST MILK

milk and milk products	wheat
eggs	nuts
fish	citrus fruits
shellfish	

The most common symptoms of allergic reaction in your baby are colic, eczema, diarrhea, and skin rashes, and the most commonly offending foods are eggs and cow's milk. If you suspect these foods or other foods are causing a reaction in your infant, you should eliminate them from your diet for at least three days and observe your baby's symptoms. If he improves, you can challenge your theory by again eating the suspect food and noticing his reaction. If his symptoms reappear, chances are they are caused by these foods. Eliminate these foods from your diet to control your baby's symptoms and to reduce the challenge to his immune system. Be sure to eliminate all sources of the offending foods in order to obtain a decisive effect.

Since milk and milk products are an important source of protein and calcium, don't eliminate them unless you are quite sure that they are causing symptoms in your infant. In this case, stop drinking milk, but try to continue to eat moderate quantities of yogurt and cheese. Since these milk products are less allergenic than milk, you may find that they do not produce symptoms in your baby. Be sure to compensate for your reduced calcium intake with calcium supplements and drink plenty of other liquids. Consult with your physician if you suspect your baby has developed a food allergy or if you feel that your consumption of milk causes a problem for your baby.

Foods, Drugs, and Environmental Contaminants

Foods and Breast Milk

Since just about everything you eat can end up in your breast milk, you need to think a little before putting things in your mouth. Highly allergenic foods are not the only ones to avoid while you are breast-feeding. Strong foods like garlic, onions, and cabbage may alter the flavor of your milk and cause your infant distress or even to reject a feeding. You should be alert to this possibility and try to identify the offending food. You may even have to hand express the tainted milk before your baby will take the breast again. The key is to pay attention to your baby and his reactions.

Some substances inhibit your milk letdown reflex. If this happens, your breasts will not produce enough milk, and your baby will be deprived of his full feeding. Some common offenders are coffee and other high-caffeine foods and drinks, tobacco, and marijuana.

Many foods have other pharmacological reactions you will want to avoid. For instance, heavy coffee drinkers may find their infants to be excitable and sleepless. Watch out for caffeine and similar compounds in coffee, tea, soft drinks, and chocolate. Don't forget that herbal teas also have various pharmacological effects. Many are no different than taking drugs, which you certainly would be wary of doing while you are lactating. Avoid all foods containing aspartame (NutraSweet). Remember that aspartame contains an amino acid that is active in brain chemistry. Very little is known about its effect on your baby's developing brain.

There are other foods whose dangers are hidden and do not cause immediate adverse reactions. Under this category fall many chemical additives, accidental contaminants of foods, and those foods implicated in the initiation and development of cancer. The effect of these substances on the nursing infant is not well understood. The infant's physiology is extremely sensitive to chemical challenges of this type so it is best to restrict your consumption of artificial ingredients and the other suspect foods discussed in Chapter 3.

Additionally, eating foods that come from potentially polluted sources should be avoided. Freshwater fish of questionable origin, bottom-dwelling fish such as sole, flounder, or catfish, or predatory fish such as swordfish and tuna might contain high concentrations of environmental pollutants or heavy metals. (More on this later in this chapter). Remember to trim all fat from meats to reduce the likelihood of consuming environmental contaminants.

Unless you are absolutely sure of the safety of your drinking water, you would be better off to purchase a bottled drinking water that certifies it is pollutant-free. Well water may contain high levels of toxic chemicals, and municipal water can contain chlorinated hydrocarbons. While the levels of these pollutants may be quite low, again little is known about their potential effects on the developing newborn. It is difficult to know whether or not your water supply is pure. In most cases, specific tests must be run to identify individual pollutants. Unless there is reason to suspect contamination by a particular chemical, the tests to verify its presence or absence will probably not be done. Drinking certified water during lactation is simply an insurance policy protecting you from unknown agents. You may want to consider this advice even when you are not lactating, for the general protection of your family.

Drugs, Environmental Pollutants, and
Breast Milk

Recent increases in the numbers of babies being breast-fed has produced an impetus for the study of drugs excreted into breast milk. In 1975, 20 percent of mothers chose to breast-feed, whereas in 1978 that figure had risen to 48 percent. It can be estimated that 50 percent of mothers breast-feed at the present time. This means that more than one-and-one-half million infants each year receive breast milk in those most important and vulnerable early months of life. Since we live in a society permeated with an ever-increasing number and variety of over-the-counter, prescription, and illicit drugs and environmental hazards such as PCBs, pesticides, radiation, and tobacco smoke, there is increasing concern for the contamination of breast milk. There can be little doubt that some of these drugs and pollutants enter breastmilk; but, because of the relative newness of the research effort and the large number of chemicals that exist, little is known about long-term, continuous dose exposure and the effects of subsequent breast milk contamination.

Research to date has produced information about short-term effects of the more common drugs and pollutants. On the average, 1 to 2 percent of the dose consumed by the mother is found in her breast milk. Because infants weigh one-tenth as much as their mothers, the amount of drug they receive from breast milk may not be insignificant. Though this varies from chemical to chemical, it is however generally regarded as a level which does not have profound pharmacological effect on the infant. There are some exceptions, however, that will be pointed out.

Fat-soluble and low molecular weight chemicals are most rapidly excreted in milk. A very large number of drugs and environmental pollutants fall into one or both of these categories and are of significance to the breast-feeding mother. Perhaps the most insidious are the environmental pollutants DDT, PCBs, and other insecticides, herbicides, and hydrocarbons. These fat-soluble chemicals are stored for years in your own body fat reserves and are only mobilized through their excretion in breast milk. Consequently, some breast milk contains levels of these chemicals that are higher than would be permissible in infant formula or other foods. Because we live in a world that is substantially polluted by these chemicals, we are all part of a grand experiment to determine their long-term effects. If you know that you have been exposed to significant amounts of these materials, you should discuss with your physician the advisability of breast-feeding. Formula feeding may be the safer alternative for your baby.

There are some things you can do to minimize the risk of inadvertent exposure of your baby to anything that can be passed into breast milk. You should avoid inhaling atmospheric pollutants whenever you can. Remove yourself from the vicinity of fumes of any kind, such as gasoline fumes, automobile exhaust fumes, paint, and other solvent fumes. Use extreme caution or avoid entirely the following activities while you are pregnant or lactating: use of paints, paint removers, and related materials, cleaning solvents, home gardening supplies such as pesticides and herbicides and any other substances that produce heavy fumes. Think about your activities and their possible dangers before acting. When in doubt, avoidance is always safest.

You must always be cautious about taking prescription or over-the-counter drugs during pregnancy or lactation, and you should always consult your physician. As in other life situations, you must weigh the benefits with the risks. However, it may put your mind at ease to know that some studies have been completed on the more common drugs, including information about the dose transmitted to breast milk and its effect on the nursing infant. The results have identified some relatively safe drugs and made recommendations for avoidance of other drugs. Those that should be totally avoided include: lithium; steroids (often used to treat arthritis and allergies); anticancer agents; radiopharmaceuticals, such as those used in certain brain- and lung-scanning techniques; sensitizing antibiotics, such as penicillin; chloramphenicol; aspirin; and all illicit drugs. Table 7.2 lists common drugs and their effects on infants. This list is not comprehensive and should not be used in place of your physician's recommendations.

Table 7.2.

COMMON DRUGS AND THEIR EFFECT ON INFANTS

Drug	Effect
acetaminophen (Tylenol)	no effect at normal doses; liver toxicity at high doses
alcohol	little, if any, effect from low doses; higher doses inhibit milk letdown and cause drowsiness, abnormal growth
amphetamines	little data, extreme caution advised
ampicillin	may cause allergies
antacids	no effect documented
anticoagulants	bleeding episodes in some infants
antihistamines	large doses reduce milk supply
anusol (rectal suppository)	no effect
aspirin	occasional dose considered safe; interferes with infant's blood clotting
barbiturates	high doses may cause hypnotic effects
caffeine	low to moderate use considered safe
cephalosporins	may cause allergies
cephazolin	may disturb infant's intestinal flora
chloramphenicol	potential harm to bone marrow; may refuse breast; sleep at feeding; vomit at feeding; anemia; shock; death
codeine	insignificant at therapeutic doses

contraceptives (oral) and synthetic female hormones	may inhibit lactation; possible breast enlargement in males; may effect milk composition
digoxin	no harm, even at high maternal doses
diuretics	may decrease milk supply
epinephrine	no harm, destroyed in infant's GI tract
erythromycin	may cause allergies
gentamicin	may cause hearing loss; kidney toxicity
gold (antiarthritic)	potential rash; idosyncratic reactions
griseofulvin (antifungal)	possible bone marrow suppression
hemorrhoidal suppositories (ephedrine sulfate, belladonna, boric acid, bismuth)	caution, no definitive study
ibuprofen (Advil, Nuprin)	inconclusive data; not recommended
indomethacin (antiinflammatory)	caution, seizures reported
insulin	no harm, destroyed in infant's GI tract
iron	no harm
Kanamycin	no harm
Kaopectate	no systemic effects
laxatives: bulk-forming, saline, or stool-softening	no harm
anthraquinone derivatives (cascara, danthron)	should not be used; harmful effects on infant's bowels

anthraquinones (aloe, senna)	problems at high doses
calomel	affects infant bowel function
castor oil, mineral oil	no harm
milk of magnesia, magnesium sulfate	no harm
lead	infant toxicity reported after use of lead acetate ointment on nipples
lithium	do not breast-feed
mercury	do not breast-feed if you have been exposed to mercury
nicotine	low dose: questionable; high dose: restlessness, diarrhea, vomiting, rapid pulse; may decrease milk supply
penicillin	may cause allergies
phenytoin (Dilantin)	uncertain
propranolol (Inderal)	no harm
steroid hormones (cortisone, prednisolone, prednisone)	extreme caution; animal studies show postnatal development retarded
streptomycin	not safe
sulfanilamides, sulfonamides	not safe in first month; caution thereafter
tetracycline	may cause discoloration of teeth, use alternate if possible
theobromine (chocolate)	OK, may cause allergies
theophylline	caution, take after nursing; irritability reported in infant

(SOURCE: Data from Platzker et al., 1980.) Adapted with permission.

If you must take medication during lactation, you can minimize the risk to your infant by adjusting your dose schedules. Once drugs enter your body, they are metabolized and, at some point in time, are cleared from your system. The longer you can stretch the time between your medication and the feeding of your baby, the less drug will enter your milk. So check with your physician and try to take your necessary medications immediately after breastfeeding.

Summary

Lactating places greater demands on your body than pregnancy. To protect yourself and your infant from certain deficiencies, you must be aware of your increased nutritional needs. In addition, you need to take some steps to insure the quality of your milk supply. In today's complex world, we can not assume that breast milk is safe just because it is part of a natural process. Here are the points to keep in mind:

1. Eat more of all nutrients in a balanced way so that you increase your caloric intake by 500 calories per day in the first three months of lactation and by 800 calories per day thereafter.

2. Be sure to get your RDA of calcium by consuming more milk products and by taking calcium supplements if necessary.

3. Increase your consumption of fluids to 2 to 3 quarts per day. Consider drinking bottled water.

4. Take a prescription multivitamin and mineral supplement specially formulated for lactation.

5. Avoid highly allergenic foods and be alert to symptoms of allergic reaction in your infant.

6. Avoid foods that are strongly flavored, contain high levels of caffeine, are artificially sweetened, colored, preserved, etc. or have been implicated in the initiation or promotion of cancer (see Chapter 3).

7. Avoid foods such as freshwater fish and animal fats that may contain environmental contaminants.

8. Take steps to lower your exposure to chemicals, drugs, additives, accidental contaminants, etc., by thinking before participating in potentially dangerous activities.

9. Take medications only under the advice of your physician and adjust your dose schedule to minimize the dose transmitted in your breast milk.

CHAPTER 7: REFERENCES

1. Committee on Dietary Allowances, National Academy of Sciences. *Recommended Dietary Allowances*. 9th ed. Washington, D.C.: National Academy Press, 1980.

2. American Academy of Allergy and Immunology Committee on Adverse Food Reactions. *Adverse Reactions to Foods*. National Institutes of Health Publication No. 84-2442, 1984.

3. Worthington, B. et al. *Nutrition in pregnancy and lactation*. St. Louis: The C. V. Mosby Company: 1977.

4. Machtinger, S., and Moss, R. "Cow's milk allergy in breast-fed infants: The role of allergen and maternal secretory IgA antibody." *J. Allergy Clin. Immunol.* 1986. 77; 2: pp. 341–347.

5. Briggs, G. et al. *Drugs in Pregnancy and Lactation*. Baltimore: Williams & Wilkins, 1983.

6. Platzker, A. et al. "Drug 'Administration' via Breast Milk." *Hospital Practice* 1980. 15; 9: pp. 111–117, 120–122.

7. Berlin, C. "Pharmacologic Considerations of Drug Use in the Lactating Mother." *Obstetrics and Gynecology* 1981. 58; 5: 17S–23S.

CHAPTER 8

Food for the First Six Months

For most of you, feeding your infant for the first six months of life will be easy. Breast milk is unquestionably the best food for human infants. It has been uniquely tailored by nature to meet all the nutritional needs of our babies and nothing more is needed for at least the first six months. It has taken more than fifty years of experimentation with infant feeding to come home to this basic understanding. From the first primitive infant formulas, which mixed corn syrup with evaporated cow's milk, to the sophisticated formulas of today, science has tried unsuccessfully to duplicate what the human body does so simply and so elegantly.

Breast milk is a complete food. It supplies all the nutrients your baby needs in the appropriate proportions for optimal growth and development, but its benefits go far beyond nutrition. It has a profound health-promoting effect. Remember that your baby is born with an immature immune system. Breast milk is his immune system for the first weeks of life as his own immunity is developing. Thereafter, as you continue to breast-feed, your baby derives immunological and other health benefits from breast milk.

Colostrum, the milk produced by the breast in the first three to six days after delivery, is extremely rich in immunological components. This yellowish, transparent fluid is very different from mature breast milk. It contains more protein but fewer calories and less sugar and fat than mature milk. The major proteins in colostrum are antibodies. These antibodies, manufactured by the mother, are an important source of immunity for the infant. They are his first defense against viral and bacterial agents and are intended by nature to protect him until his own immune system is capable of taking over. Colostrum is an extremely important first food for your baby. Even if you do not plan to continue breast-feeding, you should feed your baby your colostrum for at least three days. His immune health depends on it.

Breast milk continues to supply immunological protection to your infant even after your colostrum has changed to mature milk. The antibody concentration is now less, but it continues to be an important adjunct to your baby's immune system. For instance, if you are exposed to a new viral infection, the antibodies your body produces to defend itself are passed to your infant in your milk. Since it is difficult to avoid exposing your baby when you are sick, these antibodies will help him resist your infection and lessen its severity if he does become infected. Furthermore, if he is exposed to an infection, he can pass those germs to you while nursing, and your immune system will give him a helping hand by manufacturing antibodies for him. This dynamic relationship explains why breast-fed infants have fewer illnesses such as colds or flus than bottle-fed infants.

In addition, breast milk contains enzymes, which aid the baby's digestive process, and certain "good" bacteria, which are needed by the immature intestines. This is why breast-fed infants have a far lower incidence of colic and diarrhea in infancy and a lower risk of developing diseases such as ulcerative colitis in later life. For the first six months, your baby's digestive system is under development. The enzymes and bacterial components needed to digest foods other than breast milk are not present. This is one of the reasons why it is not wise to rush babies to solid foods. Also, human milk has a lot more cholesterol than found in cow's milk formulas. Studies indicate that this higher level of cholesterol may be needed in early life to adequately develop the enzyme systems that control cholesterol levels later in life.

It is now universally accepted that breast milk is the only nonallergenic food for infants. Not only do breast-fed infants have a lower incidence of allergic problems in infancy, they develop fewer allergies in later life. Studies show that bottle-fed babies are seven times more likely to develop allergic disease than breast-fed babies. Considering the high incidence of allergic disease in the general population, the potentially debilitating symptoms, and the poor prognosis for cure, breast-feeding should be seriously considered by all mothers as an important part of a disease-prevention program.

Formula Feeding

Unfortunately, the complexity of nature cannot be reproduced by modern technology. Formulas can approach the nutritional aspects of breast milk, but they will never be able to duplicate the immunological components. They won't be able to protect against disease, and formulas are lacking in the enzymes and bacterial components that are needed by your baby's immature digestive system. They also contain potentially allergenic ingredients.

Today's formulas have been scientifically developed to provide all the nutritional requirements of babies, and they do a good job of mimicking mother's milk on the gross

level. That is, they have sufficient protein, fats, carbohydrates, calories, vitamins, and minerals to satisfy the needs
of the growing infant. However, most formulas are made
from cow's milk. Studies have shown that the biochemical
and nutritional properties of different milks are unique. In
fact, it is now recognized that human milk contains more
than a hundred different constituents. Cow's milk does not
have the same mixture of amino acids nor the same proportions of proteins present in human milk. It does not have
the same relative amounts of milk sugar (lactose) and fat.
Its vitamin and mineral concentrations are considerably
different from human milk. In fact, cow's milk has three to
four times as much calcium and other minerals. It has been
suggested that these increased mineral levels could stress
the infant's kidneys.

All this means that you should consider the issues
before deciding to feed your baby formula, unless you are
unable to breast-feed due to adoption, illness, or exposure
to hazardous chemicals. Of course, your baby will be
adequately nourished on formula. However, he will most
likely be subjected to some nutrient excesses and some
deficiencies. Tracing these minute differences in individual
nutrient intake to health problems in later life is an extremely difficult task. We may never know with certainty
whether or not there is a connection. However, human milk
raises none of these nutritional questions.

If you are unable to breast-feed your infant, you can
still protect him from many potential problems if you are
aware of them beforehand. If possible, breast-feed your
infant for the first few days or weeks when his immune
system is particularly vulnerable and when the major portion of your immunity is transferred to him through the
colostrum. Thereafter, be very careful in choosing a formula. As discussed in Chapter 2, formulas are made of
cow's milk or soybean milk and both are potentially allergenic. Discuss your concerns with your pediatrician or
allergist.

Treat your formula-fed baby as if he were somewhat allergy-prone. You are challenging his immune system before it has sufficiently matured. To compensate, you want to reduce all unnecessary additional challenges until he has had time to adapt. Pay particular attention to signs of allergic reaction and take a conservative approach to future food introduction. Through careful feeding and an increased awareness of the symptoms of food intolerances, you can minimize your infant's risk of allergic disease.

You should take extra care to reduce your formula-fed baby's exposure to viral and bacterial infections. Without the immunological components of breast milk, his immune system is on its own at a time when it may not be able to mount an efficient defense. Protect him from colds and flus by avoiding crowds and public places particularly during flu outbreaks. If you or any other family member becomes ill, be sure to wear a mask when handling the baby, wash your hands frequently, especially before picking him up, and take extra precautions to avoid contaminating his food. And don't let grandma play with him when she has a cold! Avoid all of these unnecessary exposures. The longer you can delay the onset of infectious disease, the more prepared his immune system will be to combat it.

Vitamin Supplements

There is controversy over the need for supplemental vitamins in infancy. Breast milk, of course, meets all of the nutritional needs of our infants. But the vitamin content of breast milk is influenced by the mother's diet. If you eat properly (see Chapter 7) and take vitamin supplements while you are lactating, your baby probably does not need additional vitamins. Infant formulas have also been developed to meet the nutritional needs of infants, and no additional supplementation is necessary.

Fluoride is the only vitamin not supplied by breast milk or formula. Fluoride supplementation has been around long enough to prove its safety and its efficacy, even for infants. Your baby's unerupted teeth are undergoing mineralization in these early months of life and will benefit from fluoride supplementation. Because it is important to maintain the proper dose level of fluoride, this vitamin is available only through prescription. Discuss this with your physician. If your drinking water contains adequate fluoride, supplements may not be necessary.

Recognizing and Responding to Infant Allergic Reactions

For many babies, the first three months of life are a stressful time. Their immature physiology is adjusting to many different challenges. While it may be impossible to eliminate all the irritable symptoms, you can minimize them if you are aware of the signs of allergic reaction and know how to respond to them. As you learned in Chapter 2, foods are a frequent cause of many allergies in infants under one year. In many cases, we have come to accept these symptoms as a normal part of an infant's life. By recognizing that they may be due to foods, you have taken the first step in helping your infant to a healthier first year.

It must be noted that food allergies are not the only causes of such symptoms. If your baby develops any of these symptoms, you should consult your pediatrician. However, since many of these problems are caused by foods, your knowledge of adverse food reactions and the foods that cause them can help you and your physician treat your baby.

If you are breast-feeding your infant and he develops one of these symptoms, there is always a chance that some

Table 8.1.

SYMPTOMS OF FOOD ALLERGY IN INFANTS

Digestive problems: colic, diarrhea, spitting-up, excess gas, mucous stools.

Skin problems: rash, eczema, diaper rash.

Respiratory problems: wheezing, asthma, difficult breathing, chest rattle.

Nasal problems: stuffy nose, watery mucous, stuffiness without mucous.

Ear problems: recurrent ear infections.

Behavioral problems: irritability, difficulty sleeping.

---

food allergen from your diet has been passed to him. Review the section Allergens in Breast Milk in Chapter 7. Note any unusual food you may have consumed in the preceding three days. Some good detective work may uncover the culprit.

If your baby is formula-fed, he may have developed an allergy to some constituent of his formula. Remember, it takes time and repeated exposure to an allergen to develop an allergy. Your baby may have tolerated his formula quite well for a period of time before exhibiting a reaction. Consult with your pediatrician. You may need to change formulas, and this may involve a trial-and-error period before you hit the right formula.

As your baby grows older, his chance of developing an allergic reaction subsides. This is why delaying the introduction of solid food is a good idea. However, babies remain susceptible to these adverse reactions through their second year, so keep these symptoms in mind as you bring your baby through this transition period.

How to Know When Your Baby is Ready to Begin Solid Foods

Though breast milk (or formula) satisfies all of a baby's needs for the first six months of life, some babies may benefit from solid foods after they are four months old. You must judge from your baby's maturity; physical, mental and "digestive" maturity. If your baby is still colicky or has frequent diarrhea, he is not ready for solid foods. If he falls into the high-risk allergic disease group, he should wait until he is 6 to 9 months old before changing from breast milk to other foods. And if your baby is perfectly happy and satisfied with breast milk or formula, there's no reason to rush him into solid foods. Six months is the age recommended by most pediatricians. Check with your physician before making the change.

If your baby appears to be hungry all the time, he may be going through a growth spurt. Breast-fed babies must nurse more frequently during these times; such frequent nursing will stimulate your breasts to produce more milk. Wait a few days to see if he returns to a more normal feeding schedule. If you're worried that you may not be able to produce enough milk to satisfy him, stop worrying! It is a rare mother who cannot adequately provide for her infant and, in these cases, it is usually due to a severe or chronic maternal illness.

Sometime between four and six months of age, your baby will probably demonstrate his readiness for solid foods. If hunger wakes him in the middle of the night, he may sleep longer intervals with a small serving of cereal late in the day. If he is able to sit up with little or no support and looks interested in food, he may be anxious to begin a new phase in his life. If you are in doubt as to his readiness, consult your pediatrician and use your own best judgement. Remember, a conservative approach is the safest. Once you feel your baby is ready for solid foods, proceed cautiously and be prepared to abandon the effort for a while if your baby doesn't enjoy it or has any adverse effects.

Baby's First Meal

Generally, the best food to start with is rice cereal. Rice is hypoallergenic, meaning that few people have adverse reactions to it. Dilute one or two teaspoons of infant flaked rice cereal with your breast milk to a thin consistency. Use formula for diluting *only* if your baby is formula-fed. It is very important to introduce only one new food at a time. Never use cow's milk! As we have said earlier, cow's milk is the primary cause of allergies in infants, and its introduction into the diet should be controlled and systematic. See Chapter 9 for specifics.

Begin with a morning or noon feeding so that you will be able to observe your baby's reactions to this new food before nighttime. You may feed the cereal before nursing, at the midway point, or after nursing. Some babies are too hungry to put up with solid foods before nursing; others will be too full after nursing to bother. Let your baby decide what is best for him.

Feed him one or two teaspoonsful and watch his reaction. Give him time to adjust to this new food. He has a lot to learn. He'll probably try to suck the food and won't know how to swallow it. But soon, he'll get the hang of it. If he protests strongly or seems unable to move the food to the back of his mouth to swallow, he may not be ready for solid foods yet. If, however, he appears to enjoy this new experience and exhibits no adverse reactions, continue feeding him the same cereal, diluted the same way, once or twice a day for the next week. Thereafter, you can begin to thicken the consistency of the cereal and increase the volume (diluted volume) to one or two tablespoons. Remember, babies are very fussy about texture, so find a consistency that your baby likes. And don't feed him too much cereal. Breast milk or formula should still be his primary source of nutrition during the early stages of this transition.

Adverse Reactions

Watch your baby carefully for any adverse reactions. Though rice is considered to be a food with low allergic potential, there are examples of allergy to rice. Is your baby more colicky or does he have more gas than usual? Has he developed diarrhea or a rash? Is his breathing labored? Does he have difficulty sleeping, or is he more irritable? Check for any of the symptoms listed in Table 8.1, Symptoms of Food Allergy in Infants. Note all suspected reactions or unusual complaints. In fact, it's best to keep a diary since some symptoms appear within hours and others may not appear for two or three days. If you suspect your baby has developed one of these symptoms, immediately discontinue feeding the cereal. Observe whether or not the symptom disappears when you stop the feeding. If the symptom clears completely within two or three days, there is a good chance it was related to the food.

If your baby is under six months old, the best course of action here is to wait until he is six months old before trying again to introduce solid foods. His digestive system is not ready. If your baby is over six months and reacts adversely to this first meal, he may be prone to food allergies. Proceed very cautiously. Return to breast-feeding and consult with your pediatrician. You may try solid foods again after giving him at least two weeks to clear his symptoms. At this time, try a different hypoallergenic food, perhaps peaches. Select foods only from Table 8.2 of Infant's First Foods. Once your baby is eating a variety of hypoallergenic foods, you may reintroduce the suspected food cautiously. Chances are he will have no problem with the food at this time. (Note: Never reintroduce a food if your baby has had a violent reaction to it.)

You may begin to introduce other selected foods, pureed fruits such as pears or peaches or other infant cereals such as barley and oats. Select foods from Table 8.2. Babies under six months old should eat only these selected hypoallergenic foods. Older babies should demonstrate a tolerance to these foods before proceeding to more challenging foods. Babies who are prone to allergies should not progress to other foods until they are nine months old.

Table 8.2.

INFANT'S FIRST FOODS

rice cereal	pureed pears
barley cereal	pureed peaches
oat cereal	sweet potato
winter squash	

Introduce only one new food at a time, and observe your baby's reaction to this new food for at least four days. Be just as observant with each new food as you were with his first meal, and stop feeding the food if your baby exhibits any adverse reactions. Never introduce mixed foods. It's important not to confuse the picture. You want to be able to recognize a reaction and identify the offending food promptly.

It is wise to get your baby accustomed to all three hypoallergenic cereals (rice, barley, and oats) so that you may feed them on a rotational basis, thus avoiding potential allergic problems. Iron-fortified infant cereals are an important source of iron at this time, and he should receive two servings per day until he is 12 months old. During this time, cereals may be diluted with formula or with evaporated milk that has been diluted with an equal part of water. Remember to treat the introduction of formula or evaporated milk as a distinct food.

Homemade Baby Foods

Up to this time, you have done everything right for your baby. You have breast-fed (if possible) and adopted a conservative approach toward food introduction in order to minimize any adverse reactions. Why not continue on this track by preparing your own baby food. It's really quite simple and shouldn't be thought of as a task. If you plan properly, you can make baby food out of ordinary family meals with little additional effort. Yet the benefits are great. Homemade baby food is more nutritious because you can select only the finest ingredients and avoid overprocessing, which robs commercially prepared foods of their natural flavors as well as nutrients. And of course, it costs less, but best of all, you *know* what's in it. No fillers, starches, or sugar; no glass particles, insect parts, or pesticides. Section III of this book will give you detailed instructions for the preparation, storage, and serving of your own homemade baby food. It is designed to make the whole process easy and compatible with anyone's busy life. Give it a try.

Commercial Baby Foods

Commercially prepared baby foods are an acceptable alternative, and everyone uses them occasionally. However, you must read the nutritional information on the labels. Many mixed foods contain very little nutrition, and a lot of fillers. Infant desserts generally contain sugar, which is an unnecessary ingredient for babies. Baby food manufacturers have responded to parents by removing salt from their products. However, to keep prices down, these products do contain more water than homemade foods and often contain fillers, which have little nutritive value. Taste is another aspect of considerable difference. You will be amazed at how fresh and tasty your own homemade baby food will be. Compare its taste to a commercial product. Which one would you rather eat? After all, it's like comparing fresh-picked, lightly steamed vegetables with commercially canned, overprocessed ones.

An important key to establishing healthy eating habits is good taste. If nutritious food also tastes good, it has a better chance of standing up to the competition presented by junk foods and sugary desserts. Your baby may be deprived of the enjoyment and appreciation of nutritious foods if all he ever eats are commercially prepared baby foods.

Honey

Never feed honey to any baby under the age of one year! Honey contains bacterial contaminants that can infect your baby's intestines and has been linked to some cases of infant death due to botulism. Do not add honey to any foods or use a pacifier dipped in honey.

Summary

You should not be in a hurry to convert your baby to solid foods. Introducing solid foods before six months of age can be a big mistake if your baby is not ready. Proceed *very* cautiously, feed small portions, and do not aim for a varied diet. You will have plenty of time for that later.

Here are the key points to remember in feeding an infant under six months old:

1. Breast-feed your baby. If this is not possible, use care in selecting a nonallergenic formula and be alert to signs of allergic reaction. Never feed cow's milk or milk products to any baby under six months old.

2. Never feed any solid foods to babies under four months old. If your baby is allergy prone or still exhibiting signs of digestive distress, do not feed solid foods until he is at least six months old.

3. Introduce rice cereal cautiously, *if* your baby has demonstrated a readiness to eat solid foods.

4. If your baby has any adverse reaction to his first meal, stop. If he's under six months old, wait until he is six months old before trying solid foods again. If he's over six months old, consult your pediatrician. Give your baby at least a couple of weeks to clear his symptoms before trying a different hypoallergenic food.

5. For babies under six months old who demonstrate a readiness for solid foods: Feed *only* those foods listed in Table 8.2, Infant's First Foods. Babies over six months should demonstrate a tolerance to these foods before proceeding to more challenging foods.

CHAPTER 9

Food for the Second
Six Months

From six to twelve months of age, your baby will be in a transition period. He will go from 100 percent reliance on breast milk or formula to the beginning of table foods. This is a big jump for him! New tastes, new textures, new challenges for his digestive system and his immune system. You must go slowly and introduce new foods in a systematic manner. This chapter will give you step-by-step guidance in selecting foods that will not assault your baby's body. You will begin with easy-to-digest hypoallergenic foods and progress to more challenging foods as your baby matures and has demonstrated his ability to handle these challenges. By the end of the first year, he will be ready for *most* solid foods.

Foods for 6 to 9 Months

Once your baby has demonstrated a tolerance of the first infant foods, you may begin to select foods from Table 9.1, Foods for 6–9 Months. Until your baby is nine months old, feed only those foods listed here and in Chapter 8. If you are feeding a potentially allergic baby, proceed more cautiously, delaying these foods for two to three months. For all babies, continue to be watchful for signs of adverse reactions to new foods and stop feeding them if problems arise.

Table 9.1.

FOODS FOR 6–9 MONTHS

bananas[1]	lamb
applesauce	carrots[2]
apricots	green or yellow beans
nectarines	peas[3]
plums	apple juice
yogurt[4]	

(1) Raw, very ripe mashed bananas are generally well tolerated by most babies. However, they sometimes cause allergic reactions.

(2) Carrots contain high levels of naturally occurring nitrates. You should limit your baby's consumption to one or two servings per week.

(3) Peas are a member of the legume family, a family of foods often implicated in food allergies. Be watchful with this group.

(4) See cow's milk discussion below under Challenging Foods.

Fruits

Only the foregoing fruits should be given before nine months, and with the exception of banana, all should be cooked and pureed. Bananas must be very ripe (exterior speckled with brown spots) and thoroughly mashed. Easy methods for preparing stewed fruits are given in Chapter 12. You may also use canned fruits to prepare baby foods, provided they are packed in water or juice, not syrup. Remove fruit from the can *immediately* after opening.

Acidic foods stored in open cans have been linked to high levels of lead in children because, on exposure to air, lead is leached from the lead-soldered seams of the cans.

Vegetables

Until the age of one, all vegetables should be cooked. They will also be pureed until your baby is old enough to handle a firmer texture. After nine months, you may begin to experiment with mashed and lightly pureed vegetables and even some soft whole pieces of vegetables. Canned vegetables are not appropriate for babies since they contain salt and, in some cases, sugar. Fresh and frozen vegetables are suitable for your own homemade babyfood.

Vitamins

Now is the time (6 to 9 months) to begin giving your baby supplemental vitamins. He will begin to reduce his consumption of breast milk or formula and gradually rely more on solid foods to meet his nutritional needs. As his world expands, so will his exposure to infectious disease and pollutants. To combat these new challenges, you want to be sure his immune system is operating optimally. Good nutrition is part of the answer, and vitamin supplementation gives you that added assurance.

Liquid drop preparations should be given to your child only until he is able to handle a chewable tablet (usually around one year). Folic acid, an important vitamin for growth and development, is omitted from liquid drops because it is relatively unstable in liquid form. Liquid vitamins are available in the following configurations:

1. Vitamins A, D, and C, with or without iron.

2. Vitamins A, D, C, E, B-1, B-2, niacin.

3. Vitamins A, D, C, E, B-1, B-2, niacin, B-6, with or
   without iron.

Discuss with your pediatrician the one best suited to
your baby. All of the above are available with fluoride on
prescription. If your water is not fluoridated, you should be
giving your baby fluoride supplements to reduce future
dental caries.

After six months of age, babies have depleted their
neonatal iron stores and will need to begin finding dietary
sources of iron. Milk and milk products are poor sources of
iron. To prevent iron deficiency, baby food manufacturers
fortify dry flaked infant cereal with iron. As we have
discussed, your baby's iron requirements up to the age of
one year can be met by two servings per day of infant iron-
fortified cereal.

Water

While your infant is nursing, all his fluid needs are
provided by breast milk or formula. There is no need to
offer water except in hot weather. When he begins to eat
solid foods, his fluid requirements can no longer be met
wholly by breast milk or formula. He should be offered
water after each feeding. This will prevent him from consuming an excess of calories in an effort to fulfill his fluid
requirements by nursing. It's probably a good idea, as a
precautionary measure at this age, to give your baby bottled water that is certified to be pollutant-free. After he is
one year old, he may drink tap water if it is safe to do so in
your geographical area. However, it is advisable to have
the lead content of your water analyzed, since high levels of
lead cause mental retardation in developing children. A
1986 study by the Environmental Protection Agency esti-
mates that as many as 42 million American households may
have excessively high levels of lead in their water due to

lead service lines or the leaching of lead from the soldered seams of copper pipes. For an accurate test of the worst possible case, draw a sample of water from your kitchen faucet after the water has stood overnight in the pipes. This will assure that the laboratory test performed reports to you a measure of the maximum lead concentration. See Appendix F for additional information from the EPA.

Juices

Most people seem to endow juices with a mystical healthful quality that goes far beyond their real nutritional value. Perhaps it is because they are a reasonable alternative to soft drinks in a society that consumes 50 gallons of soft drinks per year per person. (That's a gallon per week for every man, woman, and child in the United States!) The value of juices must be put into perspective. Fruit juices *are* better than soft drinks. Juices contain some vitamins and some fiber and are therefore beneficial. However, they are not an adequate replacement for fresh, whole fruit, and heavy consumption of juices has been implicated in childhood obesity. Juices deliver a lot of calories that go down quickly and easily. They also often displace milk in a child's diet. It is best to limit your child's intake of juices. Juices can be used as an occasional treat or as an accompaniment to breakfast. Teach your child to drink water. Americans seem to have forgotten that water is a drink.

When introducing juices to your infant, wait until he is able to drink them from a cup. *Never put juice in a bottle!* Feeding juice in a bottle has been related to nursing bottle caries, a pattern of tooth decay affecting the upper incisors of very young children. Sucking juice through a nipple allows the sweet liquid to remain in contact with the front teeth for an extended period of time, especially if the child lies down. This cannot happen if your child drinks juice from a cup. The same tooth destruction can occur from giving your child a bottle of milk or formula at nap or bedtime. The liquid pools in his mouth as he sleeps, allowing the sugars to attack his teeth.

Do not introduce orange juice or other citrus juice until your baby is one year old. Citrus fruits are a common cause of allergy in infants and should not be introduced under one year.

Challenging Foods

Many of the foods that are commonly fed to infants are capable of affecting the immune and digestive systems. If your baby is not prone to allergies, you may introduce some of these foods as directed in this chapter, but be especially watchful for problems. If your baby is at high risk for the development of allergic disease, it would be safer to delay introducing these foods until after his first birthday. At that time, proceed cautiously and be alert to signs of allergy.

Table 9.2 gives a list of foods that are most likely to cause problems in infants.

Table 9.2.

FOODS MOST LIKELY TO CAUSE ALLERGY IN INFANTS

milk and milk products	wheat and other cereals
eggs	corn*
citrus fruits	fish
beef	chicken
sugar	

*Many infant formulas contain corn syrup, corn starch, or corn oil.

Cow's Milk

There are many conflicting opinions as to the best age at which to introduce fresh cow's milk to babies, though most authorities agree it should never be given before the age of six months. As mentioned earlier, cow's milk is the most common cause of infant food allergies and is a common cause of allergy in later life. Many physicians believe children should not be exposed to fresh cow's milk until they are at least a year old. Certainly, this is a valid recommendation to follow if your child is prone to allergies.

In the case of nonallergic children, readiness appears to be subject to individual variability, but due to lack of definitive knowledge, we should proceed cautiously. Milk and milk products may become important dietary sources for older children as they grow in and out of fussy eating habits. It's always nice to know that at least they drank their milk, even if they wouldn't touch anything else on their plate! Therefore, we want to avoid sensitizing them to milk.

Many babies have been started on cow's milk after the age of six months without incident. If you feel confident that your baby is not at risk for allergic disease, you could introduce some cow's milk *products,* such as yogurt and cheese, after he is six months old. If you have reason to suspect he may be allergy-prone, you should wait until he is nine to twelve months before attempting to introduce these milk products.

The best milk product to start with is yogurt. The process of culturing milk to produce yogurt renders the milk proteins less allergenic, so the risk of a reaction is substantially reduced. Also, the culture itself is beneficial in that it provides the intestines with "good bacteria" to aid in digestion. Most babies also seem to love yogurt. The texture is appealing, and they love the tartness. Select plain yogurt made from whole milk. Feed your baby a few teaspoonsful for his first milk meal, and observe his reactions closely. If he tolerates it well, feed him yogurt once a day for the next four days, and watch for any symptoms of intolerance. Chances are he will do well and love it. For variety, you can mix in some pureed fruits. Thereafter, you can introduce cottage cheese (pureed to a proper consistency) and ricotta cheese. Mixed with fruits, they make excellent meals.

As for cow's milk itself, it is best to delay introducing it until your baby is nine months old (twelve months, in an allergy-prone baby). Introduce it as you would any potentially allergenic food. Give your child a small glass of whole (3 percent fat) cow's milk once each day (preferably for breakfast or lunch) for four days and carefully note his reaction. Do not introduce any other new food while you are observing his reaction to cow's milk. Because you have waited until your baby is mature enough to handle fresh milk, he will probably have no adverse reactions. He can now begin to have milk regularly with his meals.

Children under the age of two should not be fed skimmed or reduced fat milk. The solids content of these milks is too high for their kidneys to handle properly. They also need the higher calories of whole milk. The only exception to this may be children who tend to be obese. In this case, serve 2 percent low-fat milk and encourage your child to drink additional quantities of water.

Foods After 9 Months

Once your baby reaches nine months of age, his digestive system is pretty well developed. You can begin to add variety to his diet and even start changing the texture to something closer to soft table food. Reduce the processing time for your homemade baby food and see how he likes it. He is probably also ready for some soft finger foods (see following section). Begin to choose foods from Table 9.3,

Foods for 9–12 Months. In addition, if your family has some favorite foods that are not included here, you may try them out provided they are not listed among the highly allergenic foods and they are of a proper consistency for your child to handle.

If you are feeding an allergy-prone baby, it would be best to wait until your child is twelve months old before beginning to challenge him with these foods. Be especially cautious with milk products, eggs, wheat, chicken, and beef, as these foods have all been implicated in allergic reactions.

Table 9.3.

FOODS FOR 9–12 MONTHS

egg yolk[1]	chicken
wheat (highly refined)	turkey
yogurt	beef
mild cheeses	veal
cottage cheese	onions
ricotta cheese	asparagus tips
summer squash	white potato
spinach[2]	broccoli[3]
apricot nectar	nectarine juice

Raw, ripe, mashed (no seeds or skins):

apricots	peaches
nectarines	pears
plums	avocado

(1) Egg whites are highly allergenic, and their introduction should be delayed until your child is at least 12 months old.

(2) Spinach, like carrots, contains high levels of naturally occurring nitrates and should be fed in moderation.

(3) Broccoli and other strongly flavored vegetables such as cauliflower, cabbage, Brussels sprouts, turnips, etc. are usually not well accepted by babies, but it's worth a try. Babies are individuals, and yours may like these vegetables.

Introducing Wheat

Wheat is a highly allergenic food. It should be introduced cautiously. The whole wheat kernel is difficult to digest and is also highly allergenic. For these reasons, begin with wheat products that do not contain the whole wheat kernel like white flour, white bread, and refined crackers such as Ritz or Saltines. Do not add whole wheat items until your baby is at least twelve months old. Even throughout his second year, be cautious of introducing whole grain products and granolas. They are sometimes too rough for young intestines to handle. Watch for diarrhea, stomachaches, and intestinal cramps.

First Finger Foods

In the latter part of the first year, your baby will make some pretty impressive strides toward feeding himself. He will begin to enjoy small pieces of soft table foods that he can pick up with his fingers, and will be delighted that he can eat some of the same foods as the rest of the family. This can be a very proud time for him and for you. But beware! He has now entered the age when choking becomes a real and ever present danger. You must be alert whenever he is feeding himself, and you must be careful not to feed him foods that are easily sucked into the airway. Remember, small children, even up to the age of three or four, often do not chew their food properly before swallowing.

Many parents are unaware of the foods most often responsible for choking deaths in children. Studies show that hot dogs and grapes lead the list, but there are many other potentially dangerous foods. A comprehensive list and discussion of choking foods is given in Chapter 10.

Meanwhile, when choosing finger foods for babies under 12 months, pay particular attention to texture and the size of the pieces. For instance, small children are far more likely to choke on peas than on small pieces of green beans or broccoli. Cut foods into small pieces, and *stay alert!*

Raisins seem like a natural for a soft finger food, but not only are they easily aspirated into the airway, they also often cause diarrhea, as do prunes. It is best to avoid them. Never feed babies anything on a stick! Popsicles are definitely not recommended for teething babies. Even children over age two have to be watched carefully when eating anything on a stick.

Table 9.4 will give you some ideas of finger foods for this age group.

Foods to Avoid Before 12 Months

Introduction of the most highly allergenic foods should be postponed until your child is one year old, as should the introduction of most raw fruits (other than those listed in the chart Foods for 9–12 Months) and raw vegetables. Cooking reduces the allergic potential of foods and breaks down the fiber to a more digestible form. Table 9.5 is a list of foods to avoid before your baby is twelve months old because they will most probably provoke an adverse reaction.

How to Meet Nutritional Requirements

While your baby was nursing, you had no real need to pay attention to his nutritional requirements. Breast milk or formula provided all the required nutrients in the appropri-

Table 9.4.

FINGER FOODS FOR 9–12 MONTHS

cheese cubes	macaroni & cheese
banana slices	tiny meatballs
cooked vegetable pieces	cooked apple slices
unsweetened canned fruits	fresh apricot slices
fresh pear slices	fresh peach slices
fresh nectarine slices	refined crackers
fresh plum pieces	teething biscuits
vegetable soups	arrowroot cookies
soft casserole dishes	deli sliced turkey
white toast	noodles
cheerios	dry cereals

grilled cheese or pita bread sandwiches (cut in small pieces)

Table 9.5.

DO NOT FEED BEFORE 12 MONTHS

egg white	pork
whole wheat	fish
corn	shellfish
citrus fruits	peanut butter
berries	chocolate
tomatoes	food coloring
honey	raw vegetables

ate proportions. With the introduction of solid foods, the process of weaning has begun. In the beginning, he will still be deriving most of his nutrition from breast milk or formula. Gradually, as new foods are introduced into his diet, they will begin to have an impact on his nutrition. As he approaches one year old, he may even have weaned himself completely from the breast or bottle and be entirely dependent on table foods for a balanced diet. How are you going to know if all of his needs are being met?

The easiest way to assure yourself that his diet is nutritionally balanced is to feed him servings from the four food groups: 1) Meats, fish, poultry, and eggs, 2) Dairy products: milk, cheese, and milk products, 3) Fruits and vegetables, and 4) Breads, cereals, and flours. For instance, for a seven-month-old whose primary nutrition is still breast milk or formula, this might be:

TYPICAL MENU FOR A 7-MONTH-OLD

Breakfast: infant flaked rice cereal
             pureed peaches
             breast milk/formula

Lunch: pureed sweet potato
             pureed peas
             breast milk/formula

Dinner: infant flaked oatmeal cereal
             applesauce
             breast milk/formula

By the time your baby is ten months old, his nutritional requirements are being met more and more by solid foods. His menu may look like this:

TYPICAL MENU FOR A 10-MONTH OLD

Breakfast: infant flaked barley cereal
             pureed pears
             breast milk/formula/cow's milk

Lunch: pureed lamb
             noodles
             asparagus tips
             breast milk/formula/cow's milk

Snack: cheese cubes and/or
              peach slices

Dinner: infant oatmeal cereal
              yogurt
              pureed apricots
              breast milk/formula/cow's milk

Good nutrition at this age can easily be achieved by feeding your baby balanced portions from the four basic food groups three times a day or as often as he is hungry. In addition, you may want to check that his protein requirements are being met. Adequate servings of high-quality protein (as in meat and milk products) are essential in this period of fast growth and development. For this reason, it is not advisable to give your baby a strict vegetarian diet. A lacto-ovo-vegetarian diet may be able to supply him with balanced nutrition, but it must be undertaken with extreme caution. Most pediatricians and nutritionists recommend against it.

You can determine your baby's protein needs according to Table 9.6. Simply multiply your child's weight, in pounds, by the appropriate factor and you will have his protein requirements in grams. For instance, if your child is ten months old and weighs 20 pounds, 20 × 0.9 = 18.0 grams of protein. He should eat approximately 18 grams of protein per day.

Table 9.6.

PROTEIN REQUIREMENTS OF INFANTS*

Age	Weight	Factor	GMS Protein
0–6 Months	lbs. ×	1 =	?
6–12 Months	lbs. ×	0.9 =	?

(SOURCE: Data adapted from Recommended Daily Allowances, National Academy of Sciences, 1980.)

From there, it's not too difficult to estimate his actual consumption. If your baby is still breast-feeding at will, he will regulate his intake according to body needs. If he is drinking formula or cow's milk, calculate his daily intake as follows. Milk and most milk products contain 1 gram of protein for every ounce. If he drinks three 4-ounce glasses of milk or formula each day, he receives 12 ounces daily, or 12 grams of protein. His remaining protein needs (6 grams) should be met with additional servings of meat and milk products. Most grains and vegetables are excellent sources of vitamins, minerals, and fiber, but contribute little protein. Baby food recipes in this book include estimated protein content, and most commercial preparations list the nutritional contents on the label. Read them to give you a feel for the relative nutritional values of different types of meals.

Recommended Daily Allowances are general guidelines designed for the maintenance of good nutrition in practically all healthy people in the United States. You do not need to feed your baby exactly the recommended amount each day. However, if he consistently receives less than this standard, he may develop a nutritional deficiency. If you feed more than the recommended amount, there are usually no adverse effects (other than overweight from consumption of too many calories).

Establishing Good Eating Habits

Eating habits are established early and tend to persist throughout life. Now is the time to be very strict about what you feed your child and when. Breaking bad habits is always harder than doing it right from the start. Babies rarely become fussy eaters before their first birthday and generally accept what you offer them to eat. They are more likely to be fussy about the texture of their food than the taste, unless the taste is very strong. Here are some dos and don'ts to begin right now.

1. *Never* use food for comfort, bribe, or reward. When a child needs to be comforted, give him your emotional support. Reward him with attention and activities. Do not allow food to take on an emotional aspect for him.

2. Feed your baby only when he is hungry. Don't let him get into the habit of eating just for something to do.

3. Do not use sugar or salt in his food. We develop a taste for both of these condiments. The more you eat, the more you want. And both sugar and salt disguise the natural good taste of foods. Let your baby enjoy the delicate and individual tastes of natural foods, even if you have gone beyond that appreciation.

4. Do not introduce sweet desserts until you *have* to. The time will come all too soon when he notices other children or adults eating cookies and cakes. Until that time, what he doesn't know can't hurt him. Certainly, up to the age of one year, you can conceal this reality from him. Thereafter, select sweets wisely. There are many nutritious desserts that can satisfy the sweet tooth without doing a lot of damage. See Chapter 12 for suggestions on healthful desserts. Totally denying children sweets usually sets up a rebellious state in which the child is apt to go wild at a neighbor's house or sneak to the corner store as soon as he's able to.

5. Don't insist that your child eat every bite on his plate. This kind of discipline contributes to eating problems in older children. In younger babies, it can contribute to overweight, since they are unable to tell you when they are full. Adults often overestimate a child's eating capacity. It's better to give them too little food and have them ask for more.

6. The whole family should set a good example! "Do

what I say, not what I do" won't work any better here than it does in other situations.

Good eating habits can assure your child of a healthy, happy life, and reduce his risk of developing most of the major chronic diseases. Along with good nutrition comes a healthy, optimally functioning immune system that can reduce the incidence and severity of infectious diseases. Poor eating habits can bring your child not only disease, but the devastating psychological consequences of obesity and a lifetime of battling the bulge. The stakes are high. Don't fail your child at this critical time in his life.

Summary

Your baby's transition from breast milk or formula to solid foods is critical. Here are the things you should pay attention to:

1. Start with the slow, systematic introduction of hypoallergenic foods.

2. Introduce other foods according to age recommendations outlined in this chapter. Allergy-prone babies will proceed more slowly with the introduction of all solid foods, but especially those with allergic potential.

3. Special attention should be given to the introduction of fresh cow's milk and cow's milk products such as yogurt and cheese.

4. Finger foods should be chosen wisely, avoiding those foods with a choking potential.

5. Do not feed highly allergenic foods before your baby is twelve months old.

5. Establish good eating habits *now*.

CHAPTER 10

After the First Year

❧ By the time your baby is a year old, he's ready to begin eating table foods in earnest. He's already been handling finger foods and probably junior foods. You can begin easing him into soft, easily chewed table foods, adding variety to his diet. There are still some foods you should avoid due either to their allergenic potential or the possibility of choking; but your baby is now ready to join the family for many of his meals.

If you are feeding an allergy-prone baby, you are probably relieved to be finally through the critical first year. Your cautious approach has most likely saved your infant from a lot of unnecessary distress and future allergic reactions. You can now begin to try some of the more allergenic foods on him, but proceed cautiously, feed small to moderate portions, and rotate these foods to avoid exceeding his threshold of tolerance. Be particularly careful with milk and milk products, wheat, corn, and eggs.

For nonallergic babies, many foods previously prohibited can now be tolerated. This chapter will be devoted to certain precautions, observations, or suggestions on the introduction of a full variety of table foods.

Table 10.1 includes some table foods that can be prepared with textures soft enough for babies at this age to handle. Soups and stews can be served with little or no broth, making them easier to eat with fingers. You probably have many more suggestions from your own selection of family meals. Just be sure to cut everything into small pieces and remain alert to the danger of choking.

Table 10.1.

SOFT TABLE FOODS

spaghetti and meatballs	casseroles
macaroni and cheese	soups
stews	quiche
meatloaf	pot roast
chicken pot pies	fish chowder
hamburgers	soufflés

Once your baby has demonstrated his ability to handle soft table foods, he can begin to eat just about any of the foods you normally serve the whole family. The few exceptions will be discussed in the following sections.

Choking

There are no completely safe foods. Babies seem to be able to choke on anything. It is best to restrict your child from walking, running, or playing while eating. If your child begins to choke but is able to cough and breathe (even with difficulty), chances are he will be able to clear his throat by himself. Monitor him carefully, but do not interfere with his own efforts to expel the food provided his color remains good and he is still able to breathe. If he can not clear the food completely in a few minutes, call for emergency help. He may need medical or surgical intervention.

If, however, a piece of food has completely obstructed his airway, he may be unable to cough or even make a sound. This is a very dangerous situation and requires immediate action. If your baby is off eating all by himself, you may not hear his struggle until it is too late. Therefore, always remain vigilant when your baby is feeding himself. To be fully prepared for such a situation, you should discuss with your pediatrician the course of action he would recommend. The Heimlich maneuver, in which a rapid series of thrusts is delivered to the upper abdomen to forcefully expel the food, is the usual procedure for a complete airway obstruction, even for an infant. Because this procedure carries a potential for internal organ damage, you should receive proper training from a physician or emergency medical technologist.

It is usually not advisable to remove food or foreign bodies with your fingers. This procedure has the potential of forcing the object further into the airway. However, if your child begins choking on peanut butter, it may be necessary to intervene in this way since the consistency of peanut butter makes it particularly difficult to expel. Turn him upside down and carefully sweep your finger inside the airway.

Choke Foods

Table 10.2 is a list of foods most often implicated in choking incidents in small children.

It's easy to see the danger in foods like peanuts and hard candies, but other items on this list are less obvious. Hot dogs, like grapes, seem like a good soft table food, but their roundness, texture, and outer skin contribute to the ease with which a child can inhale them into the air passages. The membranes on citrus fruit sections are often too tough for small children to chew properly. Potato chips, tortilla chips, and many dry cereals that have sharp sides

Table 10.2.

CHOKING FOODS

hot dogs	grapes
raw carrots	nuts
peanuts	hard candies
corn kernels	cherries
popcorn	peanut butter
potato chips	sharp-sided dry cereals
seeds	coconut
orange sections (membranes)	bones (chicken, fish)

can become painfully lodged in little throats. Raw carrot sticks have become a favorite snack in health-conscious homes, but they have proven to be too much for toddlers. They are among the foods most often implicated in choking deaths. It is best to avoid these foods until you are confident your child can handle them safely. There are no firm guidelines as to the age at which this will occur. You must judge from your child's ability.

Vitamins After 12 Months

As soon as your baby can handle a chewable vitamin, he should stop taking infant drops. As we have said earlier, folic acid, a vitamin necessary for proper growth and development, is omitted from liquid vitamin preparations because it is relatively unstable. The instability of folic acid also means it is often "cooked out" of the foods we eat. Choose a multivitamin and mineral chewable tablet containing an age-appropriate RDA (see Appendix A) for vitamins A, D, E, C, thiamin, folic acid, riboflavin, niacin, B-6,

B-12, iron, copper, and zinc. Iron is recommended because a good modern diet aims to reduce consumption of red meat and precludes liver (see discussion following). Be sure the vitamins do not contain artificial sweeteners or colors. If your water is not fluoridated, a multivitamin and mineral supplement with fluoride can be prescribed by your physician.

Introducing a Full Diet

By this time, your baby is probably eating three meals and two snacks a day. Throughout his second year, he will continue to expand his diet to include all of the foods you and your family enjoy. Chances are he will progress rapidly through this final transition period once he discovers the purpose for his newly acquired teeth. Remember that he is not yet ready for a low-fat, high-fiber, disease-prevention diet. Continue to feed him high-fat milk products, and do not serve him high-fiber foods until his second birthday. Here are some specific suggestions and precautions when introducing different types of foods.

Fruits

Your baby can now begin eating raw fruits provided the skins, seeds, and membranes have been removed. Apples should be peeled, cored, and cut into fairly thin slices to minimize the danger of choking. Apple seeds are poisonous, and babies are known to eat core and all. Apple skins not only cause choking, they are extremely hard to digest, and will probably cause stomach distress.

Navel orange sections can be offered if cut into very small pieces. Even then, watch carefully to see if your baby can handle the membranes. You may have to remove them, too.

You will have to judge for yourself when your baby is mature enough to handle whole, unpeeled fruits. This will probably not happen before he is two years old.

Dried Fruits

Dried fruits are not a good snack food. They are a concentrated source of sugar and because they are very sticky contribute significantly to tooth decay. In addition, they often cause diarrhea. Many dried fruit products contain added amounts of sugar or sulfite preservatives, which are known to cause adverse reactions. Don't be fooled by the "fruit" in the name. They're usually no more nutritious than candy.

Berries

Berries are still on the list of foods to avoid through the second year due to their allergic potential. When introducing berries, start with cooked berries in moderate quantity. Raw berries should not be given before the age of two, and, even then, watch for allergic reactions.

Vegetables

During his second year, your baby will begin to assert himself. The advent of the fussy eater! Suddenly, the baby who always ate his vegetables now won't touch his favorites any longer. Don't despair, he will grow out of it. In the meantime, remember that fruits and vegetables belong to the same food group. If you can't get him to eat vegetables, you will certainly be able to get him to eat fruits. Just about all kids love fruits.

You may now begin to offer raw vegetables with a few precautions. The fibers in raw vegetables are often very difficult to digest and contribute to a choking potential. You may also find your child doesn't like most raw vegetables. For instance, salads do not go over big with this age group.

Raw carrots are very popular with children. They seem like such a perfect, nutritious snack. But beware. They are high on the list of foods that cause choking deaths in children. Do not give your small children raw carrot sticks, certainly not before the age of two. You may instead give them shredded carrots or paper-thin slices, which can not break off into chunks and get lodged in their throats.

Many vegetables are rejected by toddlers because they are unappetizing, overcooked, or tasteless. Be sure to serve a variety of different vegetables either raw or lightly cooked so that they are barely soft. Cooked vegetables can be served hot or cold. Dress them up with cheese sauce, tomato sauce, salad dressings, even sour cream (for children under two).

Try mixing vegetables with other foods: quiche, macaroni and cheese, mashed potato, omelets, meatloaf, cottage cheese, yogurt, ricotta, etc. Serve them in homemade soups and casseroles.

Keep trying. Your baby probably won't reject all of them. Continue to serve him all the vegetables you are serving the rest of the family, even if he refuses to touch them. His drive to be grown-up, just like the rest of the family, may eventually win out.

Meats

You can now add pork to your baby's diet. Be sure to trim the fat from all meats before cooking. This is one habit of a low-fat diet that is fine for young children. Animal fats, as you will remember, have the potential to contain harmful chemical contaminants if the animal was exposed to them.

Some thin-sliced deli meats make excellent finger foods. Avoid the high-fat luncheon meat types of cold cuts such as bologna and salami. Plain, thin-sliced turkey, chicken, tender roast beef, and lean ham are fine.

Limit the amount of smoked meats you serve. Ham, bacon, sausage, hot dogs, and many cold cuts are preserved with sodium nitrite. For cancer prevention, it is best to serve these foods less often. Hot dogs are also high on the list of choke foods and offer little nutritional value. They are not worth the risk.

Fish

Fish is an excellent source of protein. Many types of fish are very low in fat, others are rich in Omega 3 fatty acids, those fish oils that actually protect against heart disease and atherosclerosis. Babies and small children usually reject fish. The key to acceptance is to buy only *very* fresh fish. It should have no odor of fish or ammonia whatsoever. If this is not possible due to your geographical location, try making fish chowder. It actually tastes better with "not so fresh" fish, and the milk base makes it acceptable to toddlers. Of course, be careful to remove all bones.

Children do generally like tunafish, so there's one fish you can easily serve, and it's high in Omega 3 fatty acids. Buy canned tuna fish packed in water rather than oil, to keep total fat consumption down.

A note of caution: some predatory fish like tuna, swordfish, halibut, bass, perch, and red snapper have been found to contain mercury. This is simply another good reason to maintain balance and variety in your menus to avoid over-consumption of any one contaminant. It is not a reason to stop eating these healthful fish.

Shellfish

Postpone the introduction of shellfish. Shellfish contain variable levels of microbial contamination and naturally occurring toxins, which can be very difficult for young intestines to handle. Even adults may have problems if they overindulge. In addition, shellfish are on the highly allergenic list.

Liver and Organ Meats

Pediatricians and baby nutritionists are always recommending liver for babies. It's so rich in iron! That may be so, but, in this day and age, it's also likely to be rich in pesticides and other chemicals. The liver is the detoxifying organ of the body. Most of the chemicals an animal may be exposed to in its life will end up in both the liver and the fat. Since we have no way of tracing an animal's exposure to these chemicals, we have no way of knowing if this organ meat is safe to eat. As a precautionary measure, avoid eating liver and other organ meats. They are also very high in cholesterol.

Peanut Butter

Generations of American kids have been raised on peanut butter-and-jelly sandwiches, yet little is said about the disease-promoting characteristics of peanut butter.

As we learned in Chapter 3, aflatoxins are among the most potent carcinogens known. Peanuts and corn are the two crops in this country most often contaminated by aflatoxins. Ingestion of aflatoxin-contaminated peanut butter could increase your risk of developing cancer. Furthermore, peanut butter contains peanut oil, and peanut oil is used experimentally to induce atherosclerosis in monkeys because it is unusually atherogenic. Since atherosclerosis in monkeys is very similar to the disease in man, it is a good assumption that peanut oil will also induce atherosclerosis in man.

Most commercial peanut butters are homogenized; in other words, some of the peanut oil is removed and replaced with saturated fat so that the peanut butter no longer separates on standing. This doesn't improve matters because saturated fats are also atherogenic.

Peanuts are also highly allergenic. Overconsumption can lead to allergic reactions or enhanced allergic symptoms during pollen season. Then we mustn't forget that most brands add unnecessary sugar and salt.

You can get around many of these problems and still occasionally feed your child peanut butter, but it will cost more. Many health-food stores sell natural (no salt, no sugar), aflatoxin-tested peanut butter. Check it out, but remember that peanut butter is still a high-risk (high-fat) food, and you should limit the amount you allow your children to consume.

Cereals

Dry cereals make good finger foods and snacks. But you must read nutritional labels. Cereal manufacturers have been quick to jump on the health-food bandwagon, but often the cereal they promote as "natural" contains large quantities of sugar. This is a fact with many cereals and granolas. Check the carbohydrate information on the box. Look for sucrose and other sugars; there should be 3 grams or less per 1-ounce serving. Be prepared to fight the sugar-cereal battle for many years to come because children are particularly susceptible to peer pressure and television advertising. You must also think about the choking potential of some cereals. Avoid crisp, sharp-sided pieces. They can get stuck in little throats.

Cereals are an excellent way to add fiber to a diet and, as a breakfast food, provide a combination of protein and complex carbohydrates that will carry your children through the morning without fatigue or sugar rebound effects. You should be offering your family high-fiber cereals, hot and cold, made from oatmeal, bran, whole wheat, and granolas.

Again, it is not advisable to feed toddlers a high-fiber diet. Studies do not indicate a need for high fiber in the diets of very young children, and these fibers are often too rough for young intestines. In addition, high-fiber foods are high in bulk and low in calories. Since small children have small stomachs and relatively high nutritional requirements, feeding a high-bulk diet could fill them up before they have a chance to meet their basic caloric needs. A high-fiber diet may also interfere with a toddler's absorption of essential minerals such as calcium, iron, copper, phosphorus, and zinc. Gradually add fiber to your child's diet after his second birthday.

Sweets

Chances are this is the year your baby will discover sweets. You can't hide them forever; therefore, adopt a balanced perspective toward them. Too restrictive a policy can have repercussions in future years when your child becomes old enough to help himself to candy and cakes.

Teach him the right time for sweets—after he has satisfied all his nutritional requirements, not in place of a meal and not as a snack when he is hungry. If he satisfies his appetite first with a wholesome meal and restricts sweets to dessert, he will have little room for overindulgence, yet he will not feel psychologically deprived. Healthy people who lead nutritionally balanced lives do not need to deny themselves sweets.

Choose sweets that have nutritional value, such as

fruit desserts, homemade puddings, yogurt, sherbets, carrot cake, etc. Chapter 12 will give you some recipes and suggestions for desserts which are healthful as well as delicious. Homemade desserts without fillers, stabilizers, artificial flavors and colors, and excess sugar are healthier. A small portion will satisfy the sweet tooth.

Joining the Family

By the time your baby is two years old, he is ready to join the family in a full dietary program for good health and disease prevention. The guidelines for such a program have been detailed in Chapter 6. Now, your baby can be started on new foods. The following changes can be made in his diet:

1. Substitute skim or low-fat milk for whole milk.

2. Gradually add more fiber (dried beans, whole wheat, bran, and other whole grains).

3. Encourage him to eat more cruciferous vegetables (broccoli, cauliflower, cabbage, etc.).

4. Reduce his consumption of fat, especially saturated fat and cholesterol, whenever possible.

5. Restrict his consumption of red meat. Encourage him to eat more fish, poultry, and limited amounts of lean meats.

6. Encourage him to eat fresh vegetables and fresh fruits daily.

Your success in training your child to eat properly for good health and disease prevention will depend on habits learned at home. If the family places great value on good nutrition as a path to optimal health and subsequent happiness, the child will learn from the examples set. It will be easier if you have some hard-and-fast rules regarding foods and eating habits. Children recognize the discipline in the living patterns we establish and accept them. Here are some suggestions.

Family Rules

1. No soft drinks such as soda pop, artificial fruit drinks, or other sugar-and-water concoctions. Train your children to drink water when they are thirsty, milk with meals and snacks, and juice as a special treat. There may be a special occasion or party when you allow a soft drink or two, just so you won't appear unreasonable. But be firm on this rule. If you allow on occasional soft drink for no specific reason, you have set a precedent.

2. No sugar cereals. Not even if every kid on the street has a Pac Man badge out of the box of Sugar Puffs.

3. Always eat a nutritious breakfast—something that becomes more and more difficult to enforce as your children become teenagers. No exceptions to this rule. Just accept the endless arguments you get as part of the process of your child's growing up.

4. After-school snacks must be nutritious. This is not the time for candy, potato chips, or cakes. At this time of day, most kids really need a boost of good nutrition, such as a dish of yogurt, a piece of fresh fruit, or a bowl of cereal.

5. No fast-food restaurants.

As your children grow older and are exposed to vastly different eating habits at the neighbors, the lure of television advertising, and the direct pressure of peers, the going

will get rough. After all, children do not yet have the
wisdom to eat in order to prevent premature death and
chronic disease. They just want to be like everyone else.
The best you can do is explain to them that you maintain
these rules and place so much emphasis on good nutrition
because you love them—because you genuinely care about
their well-being, not just for today but always. They may
resent the rules, but in their hearts they will know it means
you really care.

Summary

The second year is yet another year of transition. Your
baby will quickly leave baby foods and assume his place at
the family dinner table. Here are the major points to
remember:

1. Gradually introduce soft table foods.

2. Be alert to the choking potential of foods.

3. Expand the menu to include a full diet, with some
precautions.

4. Limit the amount of fiber in the diets of toddlers,
and serve whole milk products until they are at least two
years old.

5. Adopt a balanced attitude toward sweets.

6. Set some firm family rules about foods and eating
habits.

7. Progress to a full program of disease prevention
after your child is two years old.

Section Three

FOODS: PREPARATION, RECIPES, AND SUGGESTIONS

CHAPTER 11

Making Your Own Baby Food

This chapter is designed to show you how surprisingly easy baby food preparation is with the right approach and attitude. Most baby foods are simply adult foods that have been pureed to the proper consistency. For this reason, one of the easiest ways to fit baby food preparation into a busy schedule is to cook a little extra while you're preparing the usual family meal. Sometimes, this means seasoning the family's food after you have removed the baby's portion; at other times, it may mean cooking the baby's portion in a separate pan. For some foods, you will find it more convenient to make large batches of baby food and freeze individual portions for later servings. The recipes in this chapter and in Chapter 12 show you how to use both approaches to make the healthiest food for your baby.

If you're still feeling reluctant about how to fit baby food making into your already crammed life, remember this: your baby progresses rapidly through this transition time, and you will really only need to make baby food for about six months. In the beginning, your baby will have a very restricted menu, and you will need to prepare only a few foods. And, as he approaches the end of his first year, he will be eating some finger foods and soft table foods, so you really have less to prepare than you think, and there's no need to have an extensive menu.

Equipment

The equipment necessary for baby-food preparation is really rather minor. The electric food blender is by far the best piece of equipment for this' purpose. These small appliances that used to cost around $75 can now be purchased for about $25, which is a good deal, for the money you save making your own baby food will more than make up for the initial investment. You can also purchase eight-ounce blender jars to allow you to prepare small amounts of baby food conveniently.

If you already own a food processor, you can use it with the steel blade attachment to make baby foods, but you will have to work harder to achieve a smooth texture with some foods. It is also difficult to process small batches, which may limit your ability to use small portions of leftovers for baby food.

A good adjunct to the food processor is the very inexpensive hand baby-food grinder, which works just fine for small amounts of vegetables. It is not a convenient tool for processing meat or large batches of baby food, so you would not want to rely on it for all purposes.

That's about all you need for the pureeing stage. You probably already have all the equipment you need for cooking. If you do not own a vegetable steaming basket, by all means invest in one or two and use them whenever you cook vegetables for your baby or for the family. Lightly steamed vegetables retain their flavor and vitamins and are more healthful. A microwave oven is an optional piece of equipment that can be a big time-saver for a busy mother. Most of the recipes given here will include microwave, as well as conventional, instructions.

For storing homemade baby foods, you will need an ordinary refrigerator-freezer, some ice cube trays, and some zip-lock plastic bags. For reheating individual portions of frozen baby food, a microwave oven and some individual custard dishes will do nicely or an electric baby-food dish with separated food compartments. And that's about all the equipment you need. Nothing too expensive, sophisticated, or difficult to find.

Ingredients

The quality of your baby food will depend on the quality of the ingredients you select. Fresh fruits and vegetables, carefully selected and prepared, will always give your baby more nutrients than their canned or frozen counterparts. Select premium ripe produce that is free of bruises and blemishes. Remember that fruits and vegetables that have undergone attack from pests or disease are likely to contain high levels of naturally occurring chemicals that are toxic or carcinogenic. Do not risk feeding these to your baby.

When fresh vegetables are not available, frozen vegetables are an acceptable alternative for preparing baby foods. Select high quality, frozen vegetables and follow recipe directions for defrosting and processing. Some vitamins are lost in the initial processing of these vegetables, and others can be lost in defrosting, standing, and the subsequent processing procedures. Losses can be minimized if you work quickly, do not overprocess or overcook. Canned vegetables are generally not acceptable for making baby food. Most canned vegetables contain added salt and some contain added sugar. In addition, canning subjects foods to temperature extremes that destroy important vitamins (another reason why commercial baby foods are usually not as nutritious as your home-prepared ones).

When fresh fruits are not available, select canned fruits

that are packed in water or juice rather than syrup. Be sure to drain all juices, and do not allow fruit to stand in opened cans. High lead levels have been associated with acidic foods, such as fruits, that have been stored in opened cans. On exposure to air, lead is leached from the soldered seams of the cans.

When buying meats, select lean cuts and trim *all* fat before cooking or processing. Since animal fats have the potential to be contaminated with toxic environmental chemicals, it is best to keep them out of your baby food.

Preparation

Careful preparation will retain the quality of your ingredients and assure your baby of a safe and wholesome food supply. This is where home-prepared baby foods have a distinct advantage over their commercial counterparts. Because you love your baby, you are willing to pay a little extra attention to the washing, cooking, and processing of his food, so that it will provide him with the best possible nutrition.

Selecting the best ingredients is just a start. There are other points along the way where nutrients can be lost or contaminants added. For instance, overcooking can rob foods of their vitamins and their fresh flavors, as well as add the carcinogens produced as foods cook. Long delays at room temperature can increase the risk of bacterial contamination and cause the loss of important vitamins. Working with equipment or work surfaces that are not clean can add bacterial contaminants. Overprocessing in a blender or food processor can destroy vitamins, as can slow defrosting. Poor storage conditions can contribute to vitamin loss and contamination. All these variables can be easily controlled in the home kitchen to produce a final product of superior quality.

Here are some rules to follow:

1. Always use clean equipment, utensils, and work surfaces.

2. Wash fruits and vegetables carefully and thoroughly to remove any dirt, pesticides, or herbicides.

3. Wash meats to remove surface contamination. Dry and remove all visible fat before cooking.

4. To retain nutrients and to prevent build-up of carcinogens, cook all foods slowly, at low temperatures, until they are barely cooked. For vegetables, this is best achieved by light steaming. Recommendations for other foods are given with the recipes.

5. Work quickly, avoiding delays that could give bacterial contaminants an opportunity to grow at room temperature.

6. When using a blender or food processor, control processing time to achieve the desired texture and consistency in the shortest possible processing time.

7. When working with frozen foods, defrost quickly and process immediately.

8. Store homemade baby food frozen in individual portions to minimize loss of nutrients on freezing and defrosting and to avoid refrigerator storage, which can result in nutrient loss and bacterial contamination.

When preparing your baby's first foods, you will puree to a velvety smooth texture; but, as your baby grows, you can change your processing techniques to keep pace with his developing skills. After nine months, you can try reducing the processing time to achieve the consistency of junior foods. Since overprocessing has the potential of destroying some vitamins, it's best to find a texture your baby enjoys that does not require excess pureeing.

Storage

Homemade baby food should be stored frozen in individual portions. The easiest way to accomplish this is to pour the pureed food into clean ice cube trays, cover with plastic wrap and place in freezer until frozen. Unmold frozen cubes and store in a sealed, plastic bag. Be sure to label bags with contents and date of preparation. They may be safely stored for two months.

Serving

To preserve nutrients, it's best to defrost individual baby food cubes quickly, just before serving. Perhaps the safest and easiest method for reheating is to use an electric baby food dish. Just place food cubes in the individual compartments, cover, and heat, stirring occasionally until they are warmed throughout. Keep in mind that you are aiming for a temperature that is just barely warm. Babies do not like hot food, and it could be dangerous to serve it to them. Most electric dishes have thermostats, which prevent them from overheating the food, but never rely on these devices entirely. It's always best to test the food yourself first. If you use one of these dishes, you may have to allow as long as twenty minutes for heating.

Using a microwave oven is a faster method of heating food cubes, but it requires extreme caution. Foods can easily become overheated in a microwave and become a danger to your baby. Therefore, if you choose this method follow these instructions carefully and *never* feed your baby a food you have not completely tested yourself.

Microwave Instructions:

1. Place cubes in individual custard dishes and microwave on high for approximately 30 seconds per cube. Microwave ovens vary in intensity, so the time recommendations given here may not apply to your oven. You must experiment and find the appropriate setting for your microwave.

2. Stir food cubes completely and allow to sit at room temperature for at least two minutes. Stir again and test the temperature. Aim for a temperature that is uniform and just barely warm.

3. *Never* feed your baby until you have stirred the food completely and tested its temperature.

Homemade Baby Foods and Day Care

If your baby goes to day care, there's no need to deny him the benefit of homemade baby foods. Simply package baby food cubes in small, individual plastic bags (the heavy-duty, zip-lock type of bag is best). By lunch time, they will be partially defrosted, and can be heated right in their plastic bags by submerging them in hot water.

Baby Food Recipes

MAIN COURSES

Since most baby food recipes begin with cooked foods, this section will provide some *basic* recipes to get you to the cooked, basic-ingredient stage before progressing to specific recipes. These basic recipes are then used to make combination foods such as chicken and rice or veal with noodles. There is a good reason for this approach. If you've ever tried to puree meats or poultry to a texture smooth enough to please a baby, you already know that it takes more than just a blender or food processor on its highest setting. Somehow, no matter how long you process the mixture, you still end up with something rather grainy and lumpy. The secret to achieving the texture you want in a minimum processing time (remember, overprocessing destroys vitamins) is to add another nutritious ingredient that will help blend the protein fibers. The cream sauce, rice, or noodles in the recipe serves a dual purpose: it satisfies an additional nutritional requirement, and it helps achieve a texture your baby will like.

The suggestions here are just a start. You can combine your own family favorites or invent new ones you think your baby will enjoy. Just keep in mind the age appropriateness of each food selection and introduce only one new food (or one new ingredient) at a time.

BASIC LAMB, VEAL, OR BEEF

Yield: 8 oz.

*¹/₂ pound lean ground lamb,
veal, or beef*

Cook until pink color disappears. Do not overcook.

Suggestions:
- Simmer crumbled ground meat in saucepan with a small amount of water, or
- Microwave in a covered dish for approximately 3 minutes on high.

Pour off all fat.

BASIC CHICKEN

Yield: 1 1/2 cups diced chicken

*3–4 chicken breasts or
equivalent chicken pieces*

Cook chicken until tender, but not dry.

Suggestions:
- Cook extra chicken whenever you are preparing chicken for the family.
- Microwave chicken pieces in a covered casserole on high for 12–15 minutes.
- Bake, wrapped in foil, in 350° oven for 1 hour.
- Simmer with water in covered saucepan for 1 hour.

Remove the skin and fat. Cut chicken into small pieces to facilitate processing in blender or food processor.

BASIC BABY WHITE SAUCE

Yield: 1 cup

*2 tablespoons butter or
margarine*

2 tablespoons flour
1 cup milk***

In double boiler or in saucepan melt butter over low heat; add flour and stir until blended.

Cook over low heat for 1 minute while flour-butter mixture bubbles. Slowly add milk, stirring constantly to avoid lumps.

Cook over medium heat until sauce thickens.

* Use rice flour if your baby is sensitive to wheat flour or if you have not yet introduced wheat.

** Substitute formula or evaporated milk diluted with an equivalent amount of water if you have not yet introduced cow's milk or there is a suspected allergy.

LAMB, VEAL, OR BEEF AND RICE

Yield: 2¹/₂ cups or 24 cubes
Protein content: 2.8 grams/cube
Calories: 34 calories/cube
Age recommendation: 6 months (lamb)
 9 months (beef or veal)

8 oz. basic cooked, ground   *1 cup cooked white rice*
lamb, veal, or beef   *1 cup water*

Process cooked, ground meat with cooked rice in blender or food processor on high. Add water, as necessary, to achieve proper consistency.

Pour into ice cube trays, cover with plastic wrap, and freeze. Store frozen cubes in a sealed plastic bag. When serving, dilute with water or formula if necessary.

LAMB, VEAL, OR BEEF AND BARLEY

Yield: 2¹/₂ cups or 24 cubes
Protein content: 2.8 grams/cube
Calories: 35 calories/cube
Age recommendation: 6 months (lamb)
 9 months (beef or veal)

¹/₂ cup white pearl barley cooked in 2 cups water until tender (approximately 1¹/₂ hours)

8 oz. basic cooked, ground lamb, veal, or beef
1 cup water

Process cooked barley with cooked, ground meat in blender or food processor on high, adding water to achieve proper consistency.

Pour into ice cube trays, cover with plastic wrap, and freeze. Store frozen cubes in a sealed plastic bag. When serving, dilute with water or formula if necessary.

LAMB, VEAL, OR BEEF AND NOODLES

Yield: 2 cups or 16 cubes
Protein content: 4.2 grams/cube
Calories: 43 calories/cube
Age recommendation: 9 months

8 oz. basic cooked, ground lamb, veal, or beef

1 cup cooked noodles
³/₄ to 1 cup water

Process cooked, ground meat with cooked noodles in blender or food processor on high, adding water to achieve proper consistency.

Pour into ice cube trays, cover with plastic wrap, and freeze. Store frozen cubes in a sealed plastic bag. When serving, dilute with water or formula if necessary.

CREAMED CHICKEN

Yield: 2¹/₂ cups or 20 cubes
Protein content: 4.5 grams/cube
Calories: 40 calories/cube
Age recommendation: 9 months

1 cup Basic Baby White
Sauce
1¹/₂ cups basic cooked,
diced chicken

1–2 tablespoon formula or
diluted evaporated milk
(half evaporated milk:half
water)

Add diced chicken to white sauce in blender or food processor. Process on high until proper texture is obtained. Younger babies will require a smoother texture; reduce processing time as your baby grows. You may need to add formula or evaporated milk to achieve the desired consistency.

Pour into ice cube trays, cover with plastic wrap, and freeze. Store frozen cubes in a sealed plastic bag. When serving, thin with water or formula if necessary.

CHICKEN WITH RICE

Yield: 3 cups or 24 cubes
Protein content: 3.6 grams/cube
Calories: 31 calories/cube
Age recommendation: 9 months

1¹/₂ cups basic cooked,
diced chicken

¹/₂ cup cooked white rice
¹/₂ cup water

Process chicken and rice in blender or food processor, adding water to achieve proper consistency.

Pour into ice cube trays, cover with plastic wrap, and freeze. Store frozen cubes in a sealed plastic bag. When serving, dilute with water or formula if necessary.

CHICKEN WITH NOODLES

Yield: 2¹/₂ cups or 20 cubes
Protein content: 4.4 grams/cube
Calories: 33 calories/cube
Age recommendation: 9 months

1¹/₂ cups basic cooked, diced chicken

1 cup cooked noodles
1 cup water

Process diced chicken and noodles in blender or food processor on high, adding water as necessary to achieve proper consistency.

Pour into ice cube trays, cover with plastic wrap, and freeze. Store frozen cubes in a sealed plastic bag. When serving, dilute with water or formula if necessary.

BABY QUICHE

Yield: 4 servings
Protein content: 6.5 grams/serving
Calories: 110 calories/serving
Age recommendation: 9 months

2 oz. American cheese (2 thick slices)
³/₄ cup milk, formula or diluted evaporated milk (half evaporated milk:half water)

2 egg yolks, beaten

Line two individual ovenproof custard cups with small pieces of American cheese.

Microwave method: heat milk on high for $1\frac{1}{4}$–$1\frac{3}{4}$ minutes or until it almost reaches a boil. Gradually stir hot milk into beaten egg yolks and pour into custard dishes. Microwave for 9–11 minutes on medium (50%) and let stand 10 minutes to set.

Oven method: beat milk with egg yolks. Pour into custard dishes and bake 30 minutes at 325°.

Cut each quiche in half for individual serving. Remove from dish, wrap in plastic, and freeze.

FRUITS

Babies love fruits, and they're an important source of vitamins and fiber. Use fresh fruits whenever possible to insure good taste and nutritional value. The recipes here are designed to minimize your preparation time. Remember to select ripe, high-quality fruits free from blemishes. You don't want to inadvertently add toxins or carcinogens.

FRESH FRUITS: PEACHES, PEARS, APRICOTS, NECTARINES, OR PLUMS

Yield: 2 cups or 16 cubes
Calories: approximately 15 calories/cube
Age recommendations:

4 months   peaches, pears
6 months   apricots, nectarines, plums

1¹/₂ pounds fresh fruit

Carefully wash fruit. Place whole fruit in 2 quarts of water in a large saucepan and bring to boil. Boil for 8–10 minutes or until fruits are soft throughout when pierced with a fork.

Submerge immediately in cold water. When cooled, easily peel skins, discard pits, cores, and fibers, cut up and put into blender or food processor. Process on high until proper consistency is achieved.

Pour into ice cube trays, cover with plastic wrap, and freeze. Store frozen cubes in a sealed plastic bag.

APPLESAUCE

Yield: 1¹/₂ cups or 12 cubes
Calories: 15 calories/cube
Age recommendation: 6 months

6 medium apples, peeled,   ¹/₄ cup water
cored, and sliced

Microwave method: microwave apple slices in water in a covered casserole on high for 5–7 minutes or until tender. Drain and reserve juice.

Stovetop method: simmer apple slices in ¹/₄ cup water in covered saucepan until tender. Drain and reserve juice.

Process in blender or food processor on high adding reserved juice if necessary to achieve proper consistency.

Pour into ice cube trays, cover with plastic wrap, and freeze. Store frozen cubes in a sealed plastic bag.

CANNED FRUITS: PEACHES, PEARS, APRICOTS, NECTARINES, PLUMS

Yield: 1¹/₄ cups or 10 cubes
Calories: 12 calories/cube
Age recommendations: 4 months   peaches, pears
*   6 months   apricots, nectarines, plums*

16 oz. can of fruit, packed
in water or juice

Drain well. Process in blender or food processor to proper consistency.

Pour into ice cube trays, cover with plastic wrap, and freeze. Store frozen cubes in a sealed plastic bag.

VEGETABLES

Vegetables can be kept quite simple. Don't forget your baby advances quickly through the pureed food stage, and will probably be eating pieces of cooked vegetables as finger foods by the time he's nine months old.

Remember to steam vegetables *lightly* to maintain flavor and nutrients. Process them as soon as possible to avoid vitamin losses on standing and to prevent contamination. Quantities can be easily varied. For instance, you can make a whole batch at one time and freeze in ice cube trays for later servings or process smaller portions for immediate serving.

The recipes given here are representative of what you can do. They include all the vegetables you can and should introduce before nine months of age. After nine months, you will probably be serving more mashed vegetables or finger foods. If, at that time, your baby prefers the smooth texture of pureed vegetables, you can apply these processing techniques to other allowable vegetables.

WINTER SQUASH (FRESH)

Yield: 3 cups or 24 cubes
Calories: 17 calories/cube
Age recommendation: 4 months

1 medium winter squash   1 cup water

Oven method: wash whole squash and bake in a 375° oven for 1 to 1½ hours or until it can be easily pierced with a toothpick. Cut in half, scoop out seeds, and spoon pulp into blender or food processor.

Microwave method: peel, seed, and cut squash into eighths. Place in covered casserole and microwave on high for 10–15 minutes or until tender.

Process with appropriate amount of water to achieve desired consistency.

Pour into ice cube trays, cover with plastic wrap, and freeze. Store frozen cubes in a sealed plastic bag. When serving, dilute with water if necessary.

WINTER SQUASH (FROZEN)

Yield: 1½ cups or 12 cubes
Calories: 17 calories/cube
Age recommendation: 4 months

12 oz. package frozen win-
ter squash

To avoid excessive vitamin loss, defrost quickly by heating in saucepan or microwave just enough to allow repackaging into individual servings. No processing is required.

Pour into ice cube trays, cover with plastic wrap, and freeze. Store frozen cubes in a sealed plastic bag. Dilution is not usually necessary when serving.

SWEET POTATO

Yield: 3 cups or 24 cubes
Calories: 20 calories/cube
Age recommendation: 4 months

2 large sweet potatoes,   *1 cup water*
washed

Whenever possible, use sweet potatoes rather than yams because they have substantially more vitamin A and C.

Oven method: bake in 350° oven for about 1 hour.

Microwave method: pierce potato skins with fork and microwave on high for approximately 12 minutes or until tender when pierced with a fork.

Remove pulp from skins. Process with water in blender or food processor until desired consistency is achieved.

Pour into ice cube trays, cover with plastic wrap, and freeze. Store frozen cubes in a sealed plastic bag. When serving, dilute with water if necessary.

CARROTS

Yield: 2¹/₂ cups or 20 cubes
Calories: 5 calories/cube
Age recommendation: 6 months

1 pound carrots   *Water*

Wash, peel, and slice carrots. Steam over a small amount of water in a covered saucepan until carrots are tender. Reserve cooking water. Process carrots in blender or food processor adding cooking water as required to achieve the desired consistency.

Pour into ice cube trays, cover with plastic wrap, and freeze. Store frozen cubes in a sealed plastic bag.

GREEN OR YELLOW BEANS (FRESH)*

Yield: 2 cups or 16 cubes
Calories: 5 calories/cube
Age recommendation: 6 months

1 pound green or yellow   *Water*
beans, washed with ends
snipped

Stovetop method: steam over a small amount of water in a covered saucepan until tender (about 20 minutes). Reserve cooking water.

Microwave method: microwave beans with 3 tablespoons water in a covered dish for 6–8 minutes or until barely tender.

Process in blender or food processor, adding cooking water as required for consistency.

Pour into ice cube trays, cover with plastic wrap, and freeze. Store frozen cubes in a sealed plastic bag.

GREEN OR YELLOW BEANS (FROZEN)*

Yield: 1¹/₂ cups or 12 cubes
Calories: 5 calories/cube
Age recommendation: 6 months

10 oz. package frozen　　　*Water*
green or yellow beans

Stovetop method: steam frozen beans over a small amount of water in a covered saucepan, until barely defrosted. Reserve water.

Microwave method: microwave on high in covered casserole with 1 tablespoon water for approximately 2 minutes or until barely defrosted.

Process in blender or food processor, adding cooking water as required for consistency.

Pour into ice cube trays, cover with plastic wrap, and freeze. Store frozen cubes in a sealed plastic bag.

*NOTE: It is often difficult to puree beans to a texture that will be accepted by small babies. If your baby finds these vegetables too grainy, try blending them with white sauce, cooked rice, or noodles.

PEAS (FRESH)

Yield: 1¹/₂ cups or 12 cubes
Calories: 15 calories/cube
Age recommendation: 6 months

1 pound fresh peas,　　　*Water*
washed and hulled

Stovetop method: steam over a small amount of water in a covered saucepan until tender. Reserve water.

Microwave method: microwave peas with 2 table-spoons water on high for 6 minutes or until tender.

Process in blender or food processor, adding cooking water as required for proper consistency.

Pour into ice cube trays, cover with plastic wrap, and freeze. Store frozen cubes in a sealed plastic bag.

PEAS (FROZEN)

Yield: 1 1/2 cups or 12 cubes
Calories: 15 calories/cube
Age recommendation: 6 months

10 oz. package frozen peas   Water

Stovetop method: steam frozen peas over a small amount of water until defrosted. Reserve water.

Microwave method: microwave frozen peas on high until defrosted (approximately 3 minutes).

Process in blender or food processor, adding cooking water as required for proper consistency.

Pour into ice cube trays, cover with plastic wrap, and freeze. Store frozen cubes in a sealed plastic bag.

NOTE: Peas puree to a very fine, smooth texture with minimal processing and are a big favorite of young babies.

CHAPTER 12

Family Foods

Family Foods That Make Good Baby Foods

Baby-food preparation is easiest if it requires little or no additional effort. With a little thought and planning, you can prepare many family meals that can be turned into baby food. The recipes given here are just a beginning. They are intended to get you thinking about the foods you normally prepare for your family and the ingredients that go into them. You should be able to come up with plenty of family favorites that are just as suitable for baby food as these recipes are.

SOUPS

Homemade soups make wonderful, inexpensive, and delicious family meals, and they make terrific baby foods. For small babies, soups puree easily with their own broth; for older babies, they are good mashed or as finger foods if served with less broth.

Included under this heading is a recipe for popovers

that makes an elegant accompaniment to soups and provides the additional amino acids required when serving
vegetable soup. Popovers also make good finger foods for
older babies who can tolerate whole eggs.

FLUFFY RUFFLE STEW

Serves four to six
Age recommendation: 9 months (pureed)

This stew is named after the first chicken to ever grace
this recipe. She was an old laying hen who had long since
stopped laying and who had become a family pet. She was
named Fluffy Ruffles by her young mistress because her
black and white striped feathers looked like fluffy petticoats
when she walked.

1 chicken (quartered)   *2 onions*
2 celery stalks   *1 garlic clove (crushed)*
7–8 cups water   *4 peppercorns*
10 ounces frozen peas   *2 medium sweet potatoes*
1 scant tablespoon salt

Clean chicken, remove skin and any visible fat. Place
in dutch oven with 7–8 cups of water, 1 medium onion (cut
into eighths), garlic, peppercorns, salt, and 1 celery stalk
(sliced). Simmer for 1 to 1½ hours or until chicken is
tender.

Remove chicken, strain broth, and skim off fat. To the
broth add 1 celery stalk (sliced), 1 medium onion (cut into
eighths), and sweet potatoes (cut into large pieces about ½"
thick). Simmer 10 minutes.

Cut up chicken and add to soup along with frozen peas.
Continue cooking until sweet potatoes are barely tender.

Serve with bread, and you have an easy and well-balanced meal. If your baby is old enough to handle chicken pieces, he can join you. Otherwise, it's best to puree his portion.

TURKEY SOUP

Serves six
Age recommendation: 9 months (pureed)

1 turkey carcass
1½ cups leftover turkey in small pieces
¼ cup white pearl barley
2 celery stalks
2–3 carrots
Any leftover vegetables or small amounts (4 oz. each) of fresh or frozen vegetables. Best if this includes

peas, green and yellow beans, and corn.
salt and pepper
ground rosemary (use your blender if you can't buy it ground)

Put turkey carcass in very large pot and cover with water. Simmer 3 hours.

Strain broth and discard carcass. Refrigerate the broth overnight to facilitate skimming fat.

Return skimmed, strained broth to large pot and heat to simmer. Add barley, celery (diced), salt, and pepper. Simmer 1 hour. Add diced carrots, simmer 20 minutes. Add remaining vegetables and turkey pieces. Season with ground rosemary, salt, and pepper to taste.

FISH CHOWDER

Serves four
Age recommendation: 1 year

1 pound firm white fish
(haddock, halibut, etc.)
2 tablespoons olive oil
3 medium potatoes, cubed
2½ cups water
2 bay leaves
10 whole cloves
1 teaspoon sugar
salt, pepper, paprika

3 medium onions, cubed
3½ cups low-fat milk
1 stalk celery
10 whole peppercorns
2 teaspoons Worcestershire
sauce

Place water, bay leaves, cloves, peppercorns, salt, and celery in large pot with steamer basket. Place fish in steamer. Boil until fish is barely done. Strain and reserve liquid.

Sauté sliced onions gently in olive oil until transparent, but not brown.

Add cubed potatoes and onions to strained fish water and boil until potatoes are barely done. Do not overcook.

Skin and bone fish if necessary. Break into pieces and add to potatoes, onions, and water.

Add milk. Season to taste with sugar, Worcestershire, salt, pepper, and paprika. Heat, but do not boil.

Let set for several hours, overnight is best, to blend flavors before serving.

VEGETABLE SOUP

Serves six
Age recommendation: 1 year

1 16 ounce can stewed tomatoes, cut up
1/4 cup barley
3 carrots, diced
4 cups water
2 stalks celery, diced

assorted vegetables: these can be accumulated leftovers or 4 ounces each of a variety of frozen or fresh vegetables.
bay leaf, thyme, oregano, rosemary, basil, salt, pepper

Place tomatoes (including juices), water, barley, celery, bay leaf and spices in large pot. Bring to boil and simmer 1 hour. Add carrots and continue to simmer for 15 minutes. Add remaining vegetables, simmer an additional 5 minutes or until all vegetables are lightly cooked. Adjust seasoning to taste. Serve with popovers to provide all the essential amino acids.

POPOVERS

Yield: 12 popovers
Age recommendation: 1 year

4 eggs
1 cup low-fat milk
4 tablespoons olive oil

1 cup flour
1/2 teaspoon salt

Preheat muffin tin in 375° oven.

Beat eggs and milk together. Add flour and salt and beat until blended.

Remove muffin tin from oven and quickly brush cups and top surface with olive oil. Fill each cup ⅔ full with batter and return pan to oven as quickly as possible.

Bake for 35 minutes without opening the oven door. Prick each popover with a fork to allow steam to escape and serve immediately.

MAIN COURSE RECIPES

CHICKEN RICE CASSEROLE

Serves four
Age recommendation: 9 months (with white rice, pureed)

1 chicken, cut up
1 clove garlic, mashed
flour, olive oil, margarine

1 cup brown rice
2½ cups chicken bouillon

Dredge skinned chicken pieces in flour and brown in olive oil.

Coat inside of medium casserole dish with margarine. Arrange rice evenly over bottom. Strew mashed garlic around, add chicken bouillon, cover, and bake for 20 minutes in 350° oven. Arrange chicken pieces on top of rice and return to oven to bake for an additional hour or until rice is tender.

For babies under one year: substitute 1 cup white rice for brown rice. Reduce bouillon to 2¼ cups and eliminate the initial 20 minute baking time. Puree chicken pieces with rice, adding water as necessary for proper consistency.

CHICKEN BROCCOLI CASSEROLE

Serves four
Age recommendation: 9 months (see modifications below)

1 1/2 cups chicken, cooked   *2 cups white sauce*
10 ounces frozen broccoli   *3 ounces cheddar cheese*

Place partially cooked broccoli in bottom of small casserole dish. Arrange chicken meat on top. Prepare 2 cups of white sauce, add grated cheese, and cook until melted. Pour sauce over chicken and broccoli. Top with breadcrumbs and bake at 350° for 30 minutes or until bubbly.

For babies under one year: prepare white sauce with evaporated milk diluted with an equivalent amount of water. Puree baby's portion.

CHICKEN POT PIE

Serves six
Age recommendation: 9 months (pureed)

1 4–5-pound chicken, cut up   *1 clove garlic, crushed*
and skinned   *1 stalk celery*
2 1/2 quarts water   *2 teaspoons salt*
4 peppercorns   *2 small onions, quartered*
1 large onion studded with   *2/3 cup flour*
4 whole cloves   *1 pie crust*
3 carrots, sliced
2/3 cup margarine
salt and pepper
1 cup cooked peas

Add chicken pieces, garlic, peppercorns, celery, onion, and salt to water. Bring to boil and simmer for 1 hour or until chicken is tender. Remove meat from bones and cut into large pieces. Place meat in 3-quart oven casserole.

Strain broth and skim fat. Add carrots and onions and simmer 10 minutes. Strain broth and reserve 4 cups. Add carrots and onions to chicken in casserole.

Add 1 cup cooked peas.

Melt margarine, add flour, and cook for 3 minutes until bubbly. Gradually add 4 cups broth, cook until thickened. Season with salt and pepper. Pour over chicken and vegetables in casserole. Top with pie crust.

Bake 45 minutes in 400° oven.

Other Chicken Suggestions

Take a look at your usual chicken recipes. Chances are they too will make great baby food.

POT ROAST

Serves four to six
Age recommendation: 9 months (pureed)

4 pounds lean, boneless pot roast
1 cup water
3 medium potatoes, cut up

4–5 carrots, sliced
2–4 small whole onions
10 ounces frozen peas

Trim all visible fat from pot roast. Sear on all sides in olive oil to seal in juices.

Place in large dutch oven with 1 cup water. Cover and bake at 325° for 2¼ hours. Add potatoes, carrots, onions, and additional water if necessary to barely cover vegetables. Return to oven for 1 hour or until vegetables are barely tender, but roast is very tender.

Cook peas separately.

Remove roast to platter. Arrange potatoes, carrots, onions, and peas around the roast.

Pour roasting juices into small saucepan. Skim all fat. Bring to boil, add 1 tablespoon flour dissolved in a small amount of cold water and cook until slightly thickened. Serve as a thin gravy.

Older babies can probably handle this meal cut into small pieces, for the meat will be very tender. For younger babies, puree meat and vegetables with water or gravy.

Other Beef and Veal Suggestions

Beef or veal stew
Braised beef
Meatloaf

QUICHE

Serves six
Age recommendation: 9 months (see modifications below)

1 pie shell
1¾ cups low-fat milk
1 tablespoon flour
pinch nutmeg

8 ounces Swiss or Gruyere cheese
3 beaten eggs
½ teaspoon salt

Bake pie shell in 450° oven for 7 minutes. Reduce oven temperature to 325°.

Grate cheese and place in pie shell.

Combine milk, eggs, flour, salt, and nutmeg and pour over cheese in crust. Bake 35–40 minutes or until toothpick inserted in center comes out clean. Cool 10–15 minutes before cutting.

For babies under one year: mix the following separately, bake and serve with the family's quiche.

1 ounce grated Swiss or Gruyere cheese	*1 egg yolk*
1/4 cup diluted evaporated milk (half evaporated milk:half water)	

Coat a small custard baking dish with margarine. Add grated cheese.

Mix egg yolk and diluted evaporated milk and pour over cheese.

Bake at 325° for 25–30 minutes or until set.

VEGETABLE CHEESE CUSTARD

Serves four
Age recommendation: 9 months (see modifications below)

1 3/4 cups low-fat milk	*1/4 teaspoon paprika*
1/2 teaspoon salt	*1 cup vegetables (your favorite, cooked)*
3 eggs	
1 cup grated cheese (your favorite)	

Scald milk, reduce heat, and add cheese. Stir until melted. Add salt and paprika. Remove from heat and beat in eggs, one at a time.

Coat a 3-quart casserole with margarine. Put your favorite vegetables in the bottom. Top with cheese mixture.

Place casserole in pan of hot, not boiling, water. The water should be as high as the filling in the casserole. Bake at 325° for 20–50 minutes depending on the size of your casserole. Custard is done when knife inserted in the middle comes out clean.

For babies under one year: substitute diluted evaporated milk (half evaporated milk:half water) for milk above. Coat an individual custard dish with margarine. Reserve ¼ cup cheese-milk mixture. Puree 1–2 tablespoons vegetables with cheese-milk mixture and 1 egg yolk. Pour into custard dish and bake as above.

SPINACH BARS

Serves six
Age recommendation: 1 year

1 cup flour
3 eggs
1 teaspoon baking powder
10 ounces frozen spinach or equivalent fresh-cooked spinach, drained

1 cup low-fat milk
1 cup cheddar cheese
pinch salt
2 tablespoons margarine

Combine all ingredients, bake in greased 9 × 13" pan for 30 minutes at 350°.

FETTUCINE ALFREDO

Serves eight
Age recommendation: 9 months (see modifications below)

1 pound fettucine noodles   3 eggs
²/₃ cup grated mixed parme-
san and romano cheese

Cook noodles as directed on package.
Mix together eggs and cheese.
Drain pasta and return quickly to hot pan. Add cheese and egg mixture and toss until melted.
For babies under one year: mix 1 egg yolk with 1 tablespoon grated cheese mixture and add to individual portion of noodles. Puree or serve as finger food.

Other Pasta and Cheese Suggestions

Macaroni and cheese
Cheese casseroles
Noodle casseroles
Scalloped potatoes
Spaghetti or lasagne (after age one)

Just check the ingredients of your recipes. It they're on the age-appropriate list for your baby and he's already demonstrated his ability to handle them, he can eat right along with the rest of the family. Many recipes are perfectly suitable for baby food, and many others can be easily modified. If your baby can handle finger foods, you may not even have to puree them.

Healthful Desserts and Snacks

Since there is no need to serve desserts or other sweets to babies, the age minimum on all the following recipes is at least one year. The longer you can delay introduction of sweets, the better. However, there will come a time when your baby will no longer tolerate being denied something the rest of the family is served. This is when a smart approach to the sweets you offer will pay off.

Many desserts, while satisfying the sweet tooth, also contribute nutritional components. For instance, a piece of carrot cake is far better than a Twinkie cupcake, a dish of sherbet is better than a dish of ice cream. Again, the trick is to think about the ingredients that go into the recipe. What is their nutritional value? How much fat and sugar do they contain in relation to the other ingredients? Many recipes can stand to have the amount of sugar reduced considerably without adversely affecting the flavor or texture. Try it. Think about how you can modify your recipes to improve their nutritional value. Can you eliminate a frosting or heavy sauce? Can you substitute an ingredient with a lower fat or sugar content? Can you add a healthful ingredient, like wheat germ for instance. This is the approach you should take when evaluating and modifying your favorite recipes.

The other thing to keep in mind is how many sweets you are serving your family and how often. Healthy people who maintain ideal weight are not compromised by eating desserts in moderation. If desserts are served after nutritional requirements have been satisfied with wholesome foods, the likelihood for overindulgence is minimized.

PUDDINGS

Puddings are great desserts and because they are made primarily of milk; they provide all the nutritional value of milk products. Make your puddings from low-fat milk, do not top them off with whipped cream, and you have a surprisingly nutritious dessert.

RICE PUDDING

Serves six
Age recommendation: 1 year

4 cups low-fat milk
1/4 cup uncooked regular
white rice
1/4 teaspoon salt
1 teaspoon vanilla

1/4 cup sugar
1 tablespoon margarine
1/4 teaspoon nutmeg
1/2 cup raisins

Combine milk, sugar, rice, margarine, salt, nutmeg, and vanilla in a greased 1½-quart casserole. Bake, uncovered, for 2½ hours in a 325° oven. Stir often until mixture thickens. Add raisins after the first hour.

PAM'S PUMPKIN PUDDING OR PIE FILLING

Serves six
Age recommendation: 1 year

1 small pie pumpkin

Microwave method: cut pumpkin in half, cover with plastic wrap, and microwave on high for 30 minutes or until tender.

Stovetop method: cut pumpkin into large pieces, place in steamer basket, and cook in large saucepan over a small amount of water until tender.

Allow pumpkin to cool, scrape meat from skin, and squeeze out as much water as possible.

3 eggs
2 cups mashed pumpkin
1/2 cup brown sugar
1/4 + 1/8 teaspoons cloves
3/4 teaspoon ginger
1/2 teaspoon salt

4 teaspoons melted margarine
1 1/2 cups low-fat milk
1/2 cup granulated sugar
1/2 teaspoon mace
3/4 teaspoon cinnamon

Put all ingredients in blender or food processor and process on high until very smooth.

Bake in unbaked pie shell for 10 minutes at 450°, then reduce oven to 350°, and bake approximately 45 minutes. Or for pudding, pour into greased 1 1/2-quart casserole and bake at 350° for 45 minutes. Both pie and pudding are done when a knife inserted into the center comes out clean.

INDIAN PUDDING

Serves six
Age recommendation: 18 months

4 cups low-fat milk
1 cup yellow corn meal
2/3 cup light molasses
1/2 teaspoon cinnamon
1/4 teaspoon ginger
1/8 teaspoon nutmeg

2 eggs, beaten
1/2 cup sugar
1/2 teaspoon salt
1/4 teaspoon cloves
1/8 teaspoon allspice

Bring the milk to boil. Add corn meal gradually while beating with a wire whisk to prevent lumps. Allow mixture to thicken and set aside to cool.

When nearly cooled, combine and stir in remaining ingredients, pour into greased 1½-quart baking dish, and bake two hours at 325°. Serve hot. Top with vanilla ice milk if desired.

BERRY YOGURT MOUSSE

Serves six
Age recommendation: after two years

4 cups berries	*1 pint plain low-fat yogurt*
6 tablespoons sugar	*4 teaspoons unflavored*
½ cup cold water	*gelatin*

Reserve 1 cup of berries. Place 3 cups of berries in blender with yogurt and sugar. Blend until smooth.

Soften gelatin in water. Heat gently until dissolved. Stir in berry mixture.

Chill until the mixture begins to thicken. Beat until creamy and pour into serving dishes. Top with reserved berries.

NOODLE PUDDING

Serves six
Age recommendation: 1 year

8 ounces broad egg noodles	*4 apples, grated*
1/2 cup chopped nuts	*2 tablespoons brown sugar*
1/2 teaspoon vanilla	*1 teaspoon lemon juice*
1/2 teaspoon cinnamon	*2 tablespoons margarine*

Parboil noodles. Mix grated apples with nuts and spices.

Line greased baking dish with alternate layers of parboiled noodles and grated-apple mixture. Sprinkle top with bread crumbs, dot with margarine, and brown in 375° oven for 45 minutes. Serve warm.

Other Suggestions:

Vanilla, chocolate, or butterscotch puddings
Bread pudding
Custards
Plum pudding
Tapioca
Grapenut pudding

CAKES

The best way to have your cake and eat it too is to eat it without frosting. It's very difficult to make a low-fat, low-sugar frosting. Select cake recipes that do not need rich frostings to be delicious. If your family is really resistant to giving up their frosting, try topping cakes with plain yogurt that has been sweetened with a teaspoon or two of sugar or other flavoring. Or choose powdered sugar or a thin glaze made from confectioners' sugar moistened with a little milk or lemon juice instead of a rich buttercream frosting.

CARROT CAKE

Age recommendation: 1 year

2 cups sugar
1¹/₃ cups oil (safflower, sunflower, or corn oil)
2 teaspoons baking soda
2 teaspoons cinnamon
4 cups grated carrots
1 teaspoon vanilla

4 eggs
2 cups flour
2 teaspoons baking powder
1 teaspoon salt
³/₄ cup broken walnuts

Beat sugar and eggs until thickened and pale. Blend in oil.

Sift dry ingredients together and blend into egg mixture. Fold in grated carrots and nuts.

Bake in greased and floured 9 × 13″ pan in 350° oven for 35–40 minutes.

Great topped with slightly sweetened yogurt.

APPLE CAKE

Age recommendation: 1 year

1 1/2 cups sugar
1/2 cup oil
2 teaspoons baking powder
1 teaspoon salt
4 cups finely chopped,
peeled, and cored apples

2 cups flour
2 eggs
2 teaspoons cinnamon
1/2 cup chopped nuts

Mix all ingredients by hand. Bake in a greased 9 × 13″ pan for 45 minutes at 350°. Cake is best if left in pan and refrigerated.

CRANBERRY-ORANGE NUT BREAD

Age recommendation: after age two

1 navel orange
1 egg
2 cups whole cranberries
2 cups flour
1/2 teaspoon baking soda

2 tablespoons margarine
1 cup sugar
1/2 cup chopped walnuts
1/2 teaspoon salt

Peel the rind from orange and finely grate in food processor. Reserve grated rind. Process whole orange until well blended and pour into measuring cup. Add enough water to make ¾ cup liquid. Add 2 tablespoons melted margarine and the grated rind.

In a large bowl, beat egg with sugar. Add orange mixture, cranberries, and walnuts. Mix well.

Sift dry ingredients together and fold into orange mixture until well blended.

Spoon into 9 × 5″ loaf pan. Bake 1 hour at 325°.

WALNUT TORTE

Age recommendation: 1 year

4 egg yolks
1½ cups finely ground
walnuts, packed
½ teaspoon baking powder

³/₄ cup sugar
¼ cup confectioners' sugar
4 egg whites

Beat egg yolks with sugar until light and fluffy. Fold in walnuts, baking powder, and then stiffly beaten egg whites.

Pour batter into a well-greased 8″ layer pan. Bake 25–30 minutes at 375° or until torte springs back when touched lightly in center. Cool in pan.

Remove from pan, sprinkle top with confectioners' sugar. Refrigerate.

Other Suggestions:

Sponge cake
Angel cake
Banana bread
Zucchini bread
Date-nut bread

FRUIT DESSERTS

APPLE CRISP

Serves four to six
Age recommendation: 1 year

6–8 apples
²/₃ *cup sugar*
1 teaspoon cinnamon

¹/₂ *cup flour*
¹/₄ *cup margarine*
¹/₂ *cup oatmeal*

Pare, core, and slice apples into greased baking dish. Combine remaining ingredients until crumbly and spread over apples. Bake for 1 hour in 350° oven.

MELON-BLUEBERRY COMPOTE

Serves four to six
Age recommendation: after age two

1 cantaloup
1 tablespoon lemon juice

1 pint blueberries

Cut cantaloup into cubes or make into melon balls. Add berries. Sprinkle with lemon juice.

STRAWBERRY PIE

Age recommendation: after age two

1 quart strawberries

3/4 cup sugar

3 teaspoons cornstarch   *1–2 teaspoons lemon juice*
1 graham cracker shell

Reserve half the berries. Select the choicest ones and place bottoms up in a graham cracker shell. Process the remaining berries until smooth, add sugar and lemon juice and bring to boil. Mix cornstarch with a little cold water to dissolve and add to berry mixture. Cook slowly for about 10 minutes stirring occasionally. Let mixture cool. Pour over uncooked berries in shell. Chill before serving.

BLUEBERRY COBBLER

Serves four to six
Age recommendation: after age two

1 quart blueberries   *²/₃ cup sugar*
¹/₄ cup flour   *1–2 teaspoons lemon juice*

Combine berries, sugar, flour, and lemon juice in a greased 2-quart baking dish.

1¹/₂ cups flour   *3 teaspoons baking powder*
1 tablespoon sugar   *¹/₂ teaspoon salt*
¹/₃ cup margarine   *¹/₂ cup low-fat milk*
1 egg

Blend flour, sugar, baking powder, and salt. Cut in margarine. Beat egg and milk together and add to dry ingredients. Mix well. Spread on top of berries. Bake for 35 minutes at 400°.

BAKED APPLES

Serves four
Age recommendation: 1 year

4 large apples   ¹/₄ cup sugar
1 teaspoon cinnamon   ¹/₈ teaspoon grated lemon
¹/₂ cup boiling water   rind

Wash and core apples. Place in 8 × 8″ baking pan. Combine sugar, cinnamon, and lemon rind. Fill apple centers with sugar mixture. Add ¹/₂ cup boiling water to pan and bake at 375° for 30 minutes or until apples are tender but not mushy. Glaze with pan juices.

Other Suggestions:

Fruit pies (one crust only)
Fruit or berry cobblers or crisps
Fresh fruit compotes
Fresh fruit yogurt desserts

COOKIES AND BARS

OATMEAL COOKIES

Yield: about 5 dozen
Age recommendation: 18 months

³/4 cup margarine
¹/2 cup granulated sugar
1 teaspoon vanilla
1 cup flour
¹/2 teaspoon baking soda

1 cup brown sugar
2 eggs
3 cups oats
¹/2 teaspoon salt
¹/2 cup raisins

Beat margarine, sugars, eggs, and vanilla until creamy. Combine and add dry ingredients and raisins. Mix well. Drop rounded teaspoonfuls onto greased cookie sheet. Bake at 350° for 10–12 minutes.

CHOCOLATE CHIP COOKIES WITH WHEAT GERM

Yield: about 5 dozen
Age recommendation: 18 months

1 cup margarine
³/4 cup granulated sugar
1 teaspoon vanilla
1 teaspoon baking soda
1 teaspoon salt
1 cup chopped nuts

³/4 cup brown sugar
2 eggs
1³/4 cups flour
¹/2 cup wheat germ
12 oz. chocolate chips

Cream margarine with sugars until fluffy. Add eggs and vanilla, mix well. Combine all dry ingredients and add. Stir in chocolate chips and nuts. Drop rounded teaspoonfuls onto ungreased cookie sheet. Bake at 375° for 8–10 minutes.

APPLE-GRANOLA BARS

Age recommendation: 2 years

1/2 cup margarine
2 eggs
1 teaspoon vanillla
1 teaspoon cinnamon
3 cups granola*

3/4 cup sugar
*1 cup chopped, peeled
apples*
2 cups flour
2 teaspoons baking powder

Cream margarine and sugar. Add eggs, apples, and vanilla. Combine dry ingredients and add. Mix well. Bake in 9 × 13″ greased pan for 20–25 minutes at 350°. Cool before cutting into bars.

* May substitute 2½ cups oatmeal + ½ cup raisins.

Other Suggestions:

Substitute whole wheat flour for part or all of white flour in cookie recipes.
Add 1 cup granola, bran, or oatmeal to cookie recipes.
Substitute ¼ cup wheat germ plus ¾ cup flour for each 1 cup of flour.

Snacking Suggestions

Coming up with new ideas for healthful snacks is a constant drain on your creative energy, for active kids seem to have a limitless capacity to devour midmorning snacks, after-school snacks, after-play snacks, bedtime snacks, TV snacks, homework snacks, etc. Here are some suggestions for snacks for older children that will provide nutrition without excess fat and sugar.

Age recommendation: over age two

fresh fruits
melon
low-fat milk
dry cereal
low-fat yogurt
low-fat cottage cheese
cheese sticks
raw vegetables
ice milk
crackers and cheese
granola bars
nuts
sandwiches
soups

canned fruits
berries
hot chocolate made from
low-fat milk
hot cereal
frozen yogurt
ricotta cheese and fruit
low-fat puddings
fresh fruit compotes
sherbet
popcorn
trail mix
pizza

Fruits and Vegetables

To encourage kids to eat more fresh fruits and raw vegetables as snacks, make it easy for them. Kids are often too lazy to make their own and too impatient when they are hungry to wait for you to prepare them. Mix up an interesting combination of fresh fruit slices, melon balls, berries, nuts, etc., whatever is in season and goes well together, and keep a bowl of it in your refrigerator for easy snacking. Prepare some raw vegetables and store them in a plastic container filled with water in your refrigerator. Keep some vegetable dip alongside.

VEGETABLE DIP

1/4 pound bleu cheese
1/2 cup low-fat yogurt
2 tablespoons parsley
1/4 teaspoon garlic salt
pinch pepper and cayenne

1 cup mayonnaise
2 tablespoons lemon juice
1 tablespoon grated onion
1/4 teaspoon Worcestershire sauce
salt to taste

Combine and chill. Serve with cucumbers, carrots, celery, broccoli, cauliflower, green peppers, etc.

APPENDIX A

Age-related RDAs

ESTIMATED SAFE AND ADEQUATE DAILY DIETARY INTAKES OF SELECTED VITAMINS AND MINERALS[a]   (ESADDI)

	Age (years)	Vitamins		
		Vitamin K (μg)	Biotin (μg)	Panto-thenic Acid (mg)
Infants	0–0.5	12	35	2
	0.5–1	10–20	50	3
Children	1–3	15–30	65	3
and	4–6	20–40	85	3–4
adolescents	7–10	30–60	120	4–5
	11+	50–100	100–200	4–7
Adults		70–140	100–200	4–7

	Age (years)	Trace elements[b]					
		Copper (mg)	Man-ganese (mg)	Fluoride (mg)	Chromium (mg)	Selenium (mg)	Molyb-denum (mg)
Infants	0–0.5	0.5–0.7	0.5–0.7	0.1–0.5	0.01–0.04	0.01–0.04	0.03–0.06
	0.5–1	0.7–1.0	0.7–1.0	0.2–1.0	0.02–0.06	0.02–0.06	0.04–0.08
Children	1–3	1.0–1.5	1.0–1.5	0.5–1.5	0.02–0.08	0.02–0.08	0.05–0.1
and	4–6	1.5–2.0	1.5–2.0	1.0–2.5	0.03–0.12	0.03–0.12	0.06–0.15
adolescents	7–10	2.0–2.5	2.0–3.0	1.5–2.5	0.05–0.2	0.05–0.2	0.10–0.3
	11+	2.0–3.0	2.5–5.0	1.5–2.5	0.05–0.2	0.05–0.2	0.15–0.5
Adults		2.0–3.0	2.5–5.0	1.5–4.0	0.05–0.2	0.05–0.2	0.15–0.5

	Age (years)	Electrolytes		
		Sodium (mg)	Potassium (mg)	Chloride (mg)
Infants	0–0.5	115–350	350–925	275–700
	0.5–1	250–750	425–1275	400–1200
Children	1–3	325–975	550–1650	500–1500
and	4–6	450–1350	775–2325	700–2100
adolescents	7–10	600–1800	1000–3000	925–2775
	11 –	900–2700	1525–4575	1400–4200
Adults		1100–3300	1875–5625	1700–5100

[a] Because there is less information on which to base allowances, these figures are not given in the main table of RDA and are provided in the form of ranges of recommended intakes.

[b] Since the toxic levels for many trace elements may be only several times usual intakes, the upper levels for the trace elements given in this table should not be habitually exceeded.

(SOURCE: Data from Committee on Dietary Allowances, National Academy of Sciences, 1980.)

FOOD AND NUTRITION BOARD, NATIONAL ACADEMY OF SCIENCES—NATIONAL RESEARCH COUNCIL

RECOMMENDED DAILY DIETARY ALLOWANCES,[a] Revised 1980

Designed for the maintenance of good nutrition of practically all healthy people in the U.S.A.

	Age (years)	Protein (g)	Fat-soluble Vitamins			Water-soluble Vitamins		
			Vitamin A (μg RE)[b]	Vitamin D (IU)	Vitamin E (IU)	Vitamin C (mg)	Thiamin (mg)	Riboflavin (mg)
Infants	0.0–0.5	lbs × 1	420	400	5	35	0.3	0.4
	0.5–1.0	lbs × 0.9	400	400	6	35	0.5	0.6
Children	1–3	23	400	400	8	45	0.7	0.8
	4–6	30	500	400	9	45	0.9	1.0
	7–10	34	700	400	10	45	1.2	1.4
Males	11–14	45	1000	400	12	50	1.4	1.6
	15–18	56	1000	400	15	60	1.4	1.7
	19–22	56	1000	300	15	60	1.5	1.7
	23–50	56	1000	200	15	60	1.4	1.6
	51+	56	1000	200	15	60	1.2	1.4
Females	11–14	46	800	400	12	50	1.1	1.3
	15–18	46	800	400	12	60	1.1	1.3
	19–22	44	800	300	12	60	1.1	1.3
	23–50	44	800	200	12	60	1.0	1.2
	51+	44	800	200	12	60	1.0	1.2
Pregnant		+30	+200	+200	+3	+20	+0.4	+0.3
Lactating		+20	+400	+200	+5	+40	+0.5	+0.5

	Niacin (mg NE)[e]	Vitamin B-6 (mg)	Folacin[f] (μg)	Vitamin B-12 (μg)	Minerals Calcium (mg)	Phosphorus (mg)	Magnesium (mg)	Iron (mg)	Zinc (mg)	Iodine (μg)
Infants	6	0.3	30	0.5[g]	360	240	50	10	3	40
	8	0.6	45	1.5	540	360	70	15	5	50
Children	9	0.9	100	2.0	800	800	150	15	10	70
	11	1.3	200	2.5	800	800	200	10	10	90
	16	1.6	300	3.0	800	800	250	10	10	120
Males	18	1.8	400	3.0	1200	1200	350	18	15	150
	18	2.0	400	3.0	1200	1200	400	18	15	150
	19	2.2	400	3.0	800	800	350	10	15	150
	18	2.2	400	3.0	800	800	350	10	15	150
	16	2.2	400	3.0	800	800	350	10	15	150
Females	15	1.8	400	3.0	1200	1200	300	18	15	150
	14	2.0	400	3.0	1200	1200	300	18	15	150
	14	2.0	400	3.0	800	800	300	18	15	150
	13	2.0	400	3.0	800	800	300	18	15	150
	13	2.0	400	3.0	800	800	300	10	15	150
Pregnant	+2	+0.6	+400	+1.0	+400	+400	+150	h	+5	+25
Lactating	+5	+0.5	+100	+1.0	+400	+400	+150	h	+10	+50

a The allowances are intended to provide for individual variations among most normal persons as they live in the United States under usual environmental stresses. Diets should be based on a variety of common foods in order to provide other nutrients for which human requirements have been less well defined.

b Retinol equivalents. 1 retinol = 1 μg retinol or 6 μg β carotene.

e 1 NE (niacin equivalent) is equal to 1 mg of niacin or 60 mg of dietary tryptophan.

f The folacin allowances refer to dietary sources as determined by *Lactobacillus casei* assay after treatment with enzymes (conjugases) to make polyglutamyl forms of the vitamin available to the test organism.

g The recommended dietary allowance for vitamin B-12 in infants is based on average concentration of the vitamin in human milk. The allowances after weaning are based on energy intake (as recommended by the American Academy of Pediatrics) and consideration of other factors, such as intestinal absorption; see text.

h The increased requirement during pregnancy cannot be met by the iron content of habitual American diets nor by the existing iron stores of many women; therefore the use of 30–60 mg of supplemental iron is recommended. Iron needs during lactation are not substantially different from those of nonpregnant women, but continued supplementation of the mother for 2–3 months after parturition is advisable in order to replenish stores depleted by pregnancy.

(SOURCE: Data from the Committee on Dietary Allowances, National Academy Press, Washington, D.C., 1980.)

APPENDIX B
Desirable Weight Range

SUGGESTED DESIRABLE WEIGHTS FOR HEIGHTS AND RANGES FOR ADULT MALES AND FEMALES

Height[a]		Weight[b]							
		Men				Women			
in.	cm	lb		kg		lb		kg	
58	147	—		—		102	(92–119)	46	(42–54)
60	152	—		—		107	(96–125)	49	(44–57)
62	158	123	(112–141)	56	(51–64)	113	(102–131)	51	(46–59)
64	163	130	(118–148)	59	(54–67)	120	(108–138)	55	(49–63)
66	168	136	(124–156)	62	(56–71)	128	(114–146)	58	(52–66)
68	173	145	(132–166)	66	(60–75)	136	(122–154)	62	(55–70)
70	178	154	(140–174)	70	(64–79)	144	(130–163)	65	(59–74)
72	183	162	(148–184)	74	(67–84)	152	(138–173)	69	(63–79)
74	188	171	(156–194)	78	(71–88)	—		—	
76	193	181	(164–204)	82	(74–93)	—		—	

SOURCE: Data from Committee on Dietary Allowances, National Academy of Sciences, 1980.

[a]Without shoes.

[b]Without clothes. Average weight ranges in parentheses.

APPENDIX C
Nutritional Value of Common Foods

FAT AND CALORIES FROM SOME FOODS

If you choose to reduce the fat in your diet to 30 percent of your daily calories, for a 2,000 calorie diet that is about 67 grams of fat.

Food	Serving	Calories	Grams of fat
Dairy Products			
Cheese:			
American, pasteurized			
process	1 oz	105	9
Cheddar	1 oz	115	9
Cottage:			
creamed	½ cup	115	5
low-fat (2%)	½ cup	100	2
Cream	1 oz	100	10
Mozzarella, part skim	1 oz	80	5
Parmesan	1 tbsp	25	2
Swiss	1 oz	105	8
Cream:			
half and half	2 tbsp	40	3
light, coffee, or table	2 tbsp	60	6
sour	2 tbsp	50	5

Ice Cream	1 cup	270	14
Ice Milk	1 cup	185	6
Milk:			
whole	1 cup	150	8
low-fat (2%)	1 cup	125	5
nonfat, skim	1 cup	85	trace
Yogurt, low-fat,			
fruit-flavored	8 oz	230	2

Meats

Beef, cooked:			
Braised or pot-roasted:			
Less lean cuts, such as chuck blade, lean only	3 oz	255	16
Leaner cuts, such as bottom round, lean only	3 oz	190	8
Ground beef, broiled:			
lean	3 oz	230	15
regular	3 oz	245	17
Roast, oven cooked:			
less lean cuts, such as rib, lean only	3 oz	225	15
leaner cuts, such as eye of round, lean only	3 oz	155	6
Steak, sirloin, broiled:			
lean and fat	3 oz	250	17
lean only	3 oz	185	8
Lamb, cooked:			
chops, loin, broiled:			
lean and fat	3 oz	250	17
lean only	3 oz	185	8
leg, roasted, lean only	3 oz	160	7
Pork, cured, cooked:			
bacon, fried	3 slices	110	9
ham, roasted:			
lean and fat	3 oz	205	14
lean only	3 oz	135	5
Pork, fresh, cooked:			
chop, center loin:			
broiled:			

lean and fat	3 oz	270	19
lean only	3 oz	195	9
pan-fried:			
lean and fat	3 oz	320	26
lean only	3 oz	225	14
rib, roasted, lean only	3 oz	210	12
shoulder, braised, lean only	3 oz	210	10
spareribs, braised, lean and fat	3 oz	340	26
Veal cutlet, braised or broiled	3 oz	185	9
Sausages:			
bologna	2 oz	180	16
frankfurters	2 oz (1 frank)	185	17
pork, link or patty, cooked	2 oz (4 links)	210	18
salami, cooked type	2 oz	145	11

Poultry Products

Chicken:			
fried, flour-coated:			
dark meat with skin	3 oz	240	14
light meat with skin	3 oz	210	10
Chicken, roasted:			
dark meat without skin	3 oz	175	8
light meat without skin	3 oz	145	4
Duck, roasted, meat without skin	3 oz	170	10
Turkey, roasted:			
dark meat without skin	3 oz	160	6
light meat without skin	3 oz	135	3
Egg, hard-cooked	1 large	80	6

Seafood

Flounder, baked:			
with butter or margarine	3 oz	120	6
without butter or margarine	3 oz	85	1
Oysters, raw	3 oz	55	2
Shrimp, french fried	3 oz	200	10
Shrimp, boiled or steamed	3 oz	100	1

Tuna, packed in oil, drained	3 oz	165	7
Tuna, packed in water, drained	3 oz	135	1

Grain Products*

Bread, white	1 slice	65	1
Biscuit, 2½ inches across	one	135	5
Muffin, plain, 2½ inches across	one	120	4
Pancake, 4 inches across	one	60	2

Other Foods

Avocado	½	160	15
Butter, margarine	1 tbsp	100	12
Cake, white layer, chocolate frosting	1 piece	265	11
Cookies, chocolate chip	4	185	11
Donut, yeast type, glazed	one	235	13
Mayonnaise	1 tbsp	100	11
Oils	1 tbsp	120	14
Peanut butter	1 tbsp	95	8
Peanuts	½ cup	420	35
Salad dressing:			
regular	1 tbsp	65	6
low-calorie	1 tbsp	20	1

(SOURCE: Data from Human Nutrition Information Service, U.S. Department of Agriculture.)

*Most breads and cereals, dry beans and peas, and other vegetables and fruits (except avocados) contain only a trace of fat. However, spreads, fat, cream sauces, toppings, and dressings often added to these foods do contain fat.

APPENDIX D

FOOD PROTEINS CLASSIFIED ACCORDING TO BIOLOGICAL RELATIONSHIP

ANIMAL GROUPS

1. Amphibians
   frog

2. Birds (flesh and organs)
   chicken
   Cornish hen
   duck
   goose
   grouse
   guinea hen
   partridge
   pheasant
   pigeon
   quail
   squab
   turkey

3. Crustaceans
   crab
   crayfish
   lobster
   prawn
   shrimp

4. Eggs (bird)
   ovomucoid
   ovovitellin
   white
   whole
   yolk

5. Fish (representative families)
   Acipenseridae
      sturgeon (caviar)
   Anguillidae
      eel
   Argentinidae
      smelt
   Carangidae
      pompano
   Centrarchidae
      black bass
      crappie
      sunfish
   Clupeidae
      herring
      sardine
      shad
      sprat

Cyprinidae
 carp
Esocidae
 muscallonge
 pickerel
 pike
Gadidae
 cod
 haddock
 hake
 pollack
 scrod
Mugilidae
 mullet
Percidae
 perch
Pleuronectidae
 flounder
 halibut
Salmonidae
 grayling
 salmon
 trout
 whitefish
Scienidae
 croaker
 drum
 redfish
 sea trout
 weakfish
Scombridae
 bonito
 mackerel
 tuna
Serranidae
 grouper
 rockfish
 white bass
Siluridae
 bullhead
 catfish
Soleidae
 sole

Sparidae
 porgy
 red snapper
Stolephoridae
 anchovy
Xyphidae
 swordfish

6. Red Meats (flesh and internal organs)
 a. Bovidae
  Cow
   beef
   calf
   steer
   veal
  Gelatin
  Goat
  Ox
  Sheep
   lamb
   mutton
  Sweetbread
 b. Suidae (pig)
  bacon
  boar
  ham
  hog
  pig
  pork
  sausage
  scrapple
  sow
  swine

7. Milk Products (cow, goat)
  butter
  buttermilk
  casein
  cheese
  cream
   sour
   whipped

ice cream
lactalbumin
milk
  condensed
  evaporated
  homogenized
  powdered
  raw
  skimmed
selected infant formulas
yogurt

8. Mollusks
  abalone
  clam
  cockle
  mussel
  octopus
  oyster
  quahog
  scallop
  snail (escargot)
  squid

9. Reptiles
  alligator
  crocodile
  rattlesnake
  terrapin
  turtle

PLANT GROUPS

10. Apple family
  apple
    cider
    vinegar (apple cider)
  crabapple
  pear
  quince
  quince seed

11. Banana family
  banana
  plantain

12. Beech family
  beechnut
  chestnut
  chinquapin

13. Birch family
  filbert
  hazelnut
  wintergreen (*Betula* spp.)

14. Buckwheat family
  buckwheat
  rhubarb
  sorrel

15. Cashew family
  cashew
  mango
  pistachio

16. Citrus family
  citron
  grapefruit
  kumquat
  lemon
  lime
  orange
  tangelo
  tangerine

17. Cola nut family
  chocolate (cocoa)
  cola (kola) nut

18. Fungi
  mushroom
  truffle
  yeast
    baker's

brewer's
distiller's
Fleischmann's
lactose-fermenting
lager beer

19. Ginger family
    cardamon (cardamom,
cardamum)
    East Indian arrowroot
    ginger
    turmeric

20. Goosefoot family
    beet
    lamb's quarters
    spinach
    Swiss chard

21. Gourd (melon) family
    cantaloup (muskmelon)
    casaba (winter muskmelon)
    Chinese watermelon
    citron melon
    cucumber
    gherkin
    honeydew melon
    Persian melon
    pumpkin
    summer squash
    watermelon
    winter squash

22. Grape family
    champagne
    grape
    raisin
    vinegar (wine)
    wine (grape)

23. Grass (cereal) family
    bamboo
    barley

corn (maize)
hominy
malt (germinated grain)
millet
oat
popcorn
rice
rye
sorghum
sugar cane
wheat
    bran
    germ
    gliadin
    globulin
    glutenin
    leucosin
    proteose
    whole

24. Heath family
    black huckleberry
    blueberry
    cranberry
    wintergreen (*Pyrola* spp.)

25. Laurel family
    avocado
    bay leaf
    cinnamon
    sassafras

26. Lecythis family
    Brazil nut

27. Lily family
    aloe
    asparagus
    chives
    garlic
    leek
    onion

sarsaparilla
shallot

28. Madder family
    coffee

29. Mallow family
    cottonseed
    marshmallow
    okra (gumbo)

30. Mint family
    balm
    basil
    catnip
    horehound
    Japanese artichoke
    lavender
    marjoram
    mint
    oregano
    peppermint
    rosemary
    sage
    savory
    spearmint
    thyme

31. Morning glory family
    sweet potato
    yam

32. Mulberry family
    breadfruit
    breadnut
    fig
    hop

33. Mustard family
    broccoli
    Brussels sprouts
    cabbage
    cauliflower

collards
garden cress
horseradish
kale
kohlrabi
mustard
radish
rutabaga
turnip
watercress

34. Myrtle family
    allspice
    clove
    guava
    myrtle
    pimento

35. Nightshade family
    bell pepper
    cayenne pepper
    chili (paprika) (red pepper)
    eggplant
    ground cherry
    melon pear
    potato (white)
    strawberry tomato
    tobacco
    tomato
    tree tomato

36. Nutmeg family
    mace
    nutmeg

37. Olive family
    jasmine
    olive

38. Orchid family
    vanilla

39. Palm family
    cabbage palm

coconut
date

40. Papaya family
   papain
   papaya

41. Parsley family
   anise
   caraway
   carrot
   celeriac
   celery
   coriander
   dill
   fennel
   parsley
   parsnip

42. Pea (legume) family
   acacia
   alfalfa
   black-eyed pea (cowpea)
   broad bean (fava bean)
   carob bean (St. John's bread)
   chick pea (garbanzo)
   common bean
     kidney
     navy
     pinto
     string (green)
   Jack bean
   lentil
   licorice
   lima bean
   mesquite
   pea
   peanut
   soybean
   tamarind
   tragacanth

43. Pepper family
   black pepper

44. Pine family
   juniper
   pine nut (pignolia)

45. Pineapple family
   pineapple

46. Plum family
   almond
   apricot
   cherry
   peach, nectarine
   plum, prune

47. Poppy family
   poppyseed

48. Rose family
   black raspberry
   blackberry
   boysenberry, dewberry, loganberry
   red raspberry
   strawberry

49. Saxifrage family
   currant, gooseberry

50. Sunflower (composite, aster) family
   absinthe (sagebrush, wormwood)
   artichoke
   camomile
   chicory
   dandelion
   endive, escarole
   Jerusalem artichoke
   lettuce

oyster plant (salsify)   52. Walnut family
safflower   black walnut
sunflower seed   butternut
tansy   English walnut
tarragon   hickory nut
                                     pecan
51. Tea family
tea

(SOURCE: Data from American Academy of Allergy and Immunology Committee on Adverse Food Reactions, National Institutes of Health Publication No. 84-2442, 1984.)

APPENDIX E

FOOD ADDITIVES THAT CAUSE ALLERGIES

Additive	Use/Source in Diet
tartrazine (FD&C yellow #5)	food coloring
erythrosin	food coloring
amaranth (FD&C red #2)	food coloring
metabisulfite	preservative
sulfur dioxide	preservative
BHA/BHT	preservative
propylgallate	preservative
sodium nitrite	preservative
sodium benzoate	preservative
monosodium glutamate	flavoring
quinine	flavoring
menthol	flavoring
saccharin	artificial sweetener
aspartame (NutraSweet)	artificial sweetener

(SOURCE: Data from Moneret-Vautrin D. A. "Food, antigens, and additives" *J. Allergy Clin. Immunol.*, Vol. 75; 5:pp. 1039–1046, 1986.)

FOOD ADDITIVES SUSPECTED OF CAUSING CANCER IN LABORATORY ANIMALS

Additive	Use/Source in Diet
cyclamate	artificial sweetener
saccharin	artificial sweetener
dulcin	artificial sweetener
xylitol	sweetener
sucrose	sweetener
amaranth (FD&C red #2)	food coloring
FD&C red #32	food coloring
FD&C orange #2	food coloring
butter yellow (N,N-dimethyl-4-aminoazobenzene)	food coloring
safrole	flavoring
oil of calamus	flavoring
cinnamyl anthranilate	flavoring
diethylpyrocarbonate	preservative
8-hydroxyquinoline	preservative
BHT (butylated hydroxytoluene)	preservative
trichloroethylene	extractant
carrageenin	emulsifier
myrj 45 (polyoxyethylene monostearate)	antistaling agent
tannic acid	wine, fruits
tween-60 (sorbitan monostearate)	antibloom agent in chocolates
carboxymethylcellulose	ice cream stabilizer

(SOURCE: Committee on Diet, Nutrition, and Cancer, National Academy of Sciences, 1982.)

APPENDIX F

SUGGESTED READING AND SOURCES OF INFORMATION

1. Committee on Dietary Allowances, National Academy of Sciences. *Recommended Dietary Allowances*, 9th ed., Washington, D.C.: National Academy Press, 1980.

2. *Diet, Nutrition and Cancer Prevention*, U.S. Department of Health and Human Services, NIH Publication no. 85-2711, 1984. Available free of charge from the American Cancer Society at 1-800-4-CANCER.

3. American Heart Association, *1986 Heart Facts*, Dallas, TX, 1986. Available free of charge from your state affiliate, or call 214-373-6300.

4. Rapp, Doris J., *Allergies and Your Family*, New York: Sterling Publishing Co., 1985.

5. La Leche League International, *The Womanly Art of Breastfeeding*, 3rd ed., New York: Plume, 1983.

6. Huggins, Kathleen, *The Nursing Mother's Companion*, Boston: Harvard Common Press, 1986.

7. Eiger, Marvin S., M.D., and Olds, Sally Wendkos, *The Complete Book of Breastfeeding*, New York: Workman Publishing, 1987.

8. Environmental Protection Agency Citizens Handbook, *Lead in Drinking Water, Should You Be Concerned?*, available free of charge from the U. S. Environmental Protection Agency, 401 M Street SW, Washington, D.C. 20460.

9. Morash, Marian, *The Victory Garden Cookbook,* New York: Alfred A. Knopf, 1982.

10. Better Homes and Gardens, *All-Time Favorite Vegetable Recipes,* Des Moines: Meredith Corporation, 1977.

11. Better Homes and Gardens, *Microwave Vegetables,* Des Moines, Meredith Corporation, 1986.

12. DeBakey, Michael et al., *The Living Heart Diet,* New York: Raven Press Books, Inc., 1986.

13. *The American Heart Association Cook Book,* New York: Ballantine Books, 1973.

14. Brody, Jane, *Good Food Book: Living the High Carbohydrate Way,* New York: Bantam Books, Inc., 1985.

15. Nutrition Action Health Letter is available by subscription from the non-profit Center for Science in the Public Interest, 1501 16th Street NW, Washington, D.C. 20036.

16. Tufts University Diet and Nutrition Letter is available by subscription from 475 Park Avenue S, New York, NY 10016.

17. The Harvard Medical School Health Letter is available by subscription from 79 Garden Street, Cambridge, MA 02138.

RECIPE INDEX

GENERAL INDEX

Additives. *See* Food additives
Aflatoxins, 57
Aging, causes of, 51
Allergens, 29, 123–125
Allergies. *See also under specific*
type of food or allergy
  cyclic food, 40
  development of, 31
  fixed food, 39–40
  food additives and, 248–249
  heredity and, 29
  highly allergenic foods, 39,
    114–115
  lifelong, 30
  masked food, 40–41
  treatments for, 30, 43–44
Allergies, infants and
  breast milk and, 34
  cow's milk and, 34, 36
  diarrhea and, 36
  early feeding and, 31–32, 33
  formulas and, 33–35
  heredity and, 29
  how to prevent, 33–36
  pets and, 35
  solid foods and, 33–34, 35, 154
  soybean formulas and, 34–35
  symptoms of, 33, 140–141
Allergies to food, after age one,
  37–39
  cow's milk and, 42–43

cyclic food, 40
fixed food, 39–40
highly allergenic foods, 39, 154
how to prevent, 41–42
masked food, 40–41
symptoms of, 38
types of, 39–41
American Academy of Pediatrics,
  xiii–xiv, 83, 84, 85
American Cancer Society, xiv
American Heart Association, xiv,
  4
Amino acids
  description of, 7
  sources of, 21
Animal proteins, importance of,
  21
Applesauce, used to control
  diarrhea, 36
Artificial sweetners, allergic
  reactions to, 47, 248, 249
Aspartame. *See* NutraSweet
Asthma, 28
  infant food allergies and, 32
  flavorings and, 46
  food colorings and, 46
  preservatives and, 46
Atherosclerosis
  carbohydrates and, 77
  causes of, 69–79
  cholesterol and, 72

development of, 70–71
fats and, 71–77
fiber and, 77
foods that increase the risk of,
    75
genetic factors and, 70
hyperlipidemia and, 72
lipoproteins and, 72–73
minerals and, 77
olive oil and, 55
Omega 3 oils and, 75–77
plaque formation and, 70–71
in young children, 69
Azo dyes, allergic reactions to, 46

Banana
    for 6–12 month old, 150
    used to control diarrhea, 36
Behavioral problems
    food colorings and, 45
    sugar and, 88
Berries, 171
Beta-carotene, 14, 60–61, 112
BHA/BHT
    allergic reactions to, 46, 248
    cancer and, 59, 249
Biotin
    importance of, 13
    sources of, 13
Birth defects, selenium and, 63
Breast-feeding. *See* Lactation
Breast milk. *See also* Lactation
    allergens in, 123–125
    allergies and, 34
    benefits of, 118, 135–137
    cholesterol in, 137
    effects of drugs and environ-
        mental pollutants in, 127–133
    effects of foods in, 126–127
    fat content in, 65

Calcium
    hypertension and, 96
    importance of, 15, 16, 17
    kidney stones and, 96
    lactation and, 17, 123
    osteoporosis and, 97–98

pregnancy and, 17
sources of, 16, 17, 21, 113
Caloric requirements, 6
Cancer
    alcoholism and, 49
    causes of, 49
    cooking of food and, 59–60
    cruciferous vegetables and, 64
    development of, 50–52
    diet and, xv, 49–67
    fat and, 54–56
    fiber and, 63–64
    food additives and, 59, 249
    food colorings and, 45, 249
    foods known to contain
        cancer-promoting chemicals,
        58
    initiation and, 51–52
    molds and, 57–58
    obesity and, 52
    preventive measures in infants
        and, 64–66
    promotion and, 52
    salt-cured, smoked or pickled
        foods and, 56
    selenium and, 62–63
    smoking and, xv, 49, 50
    vitamin A and, 60–61
    vitamin C and, 61–62
    vitamin E and, 62
Carbohydrates
    atherosclerosis and, 77
    sources of, 8, 21
Cardiovascular disease. *See*
    Coronary heart disease
Cereals, introducing, 143,
    145–146, 175–176
Cheese
    allergies and, 42
    for 6–12 month old, 155
Chloride, importance of, 18
Choking, 158–159, 167–169, 172
Cholesterol
    atherosclerosis and, 72
    in breast milk, 137
    cancer and, 55
    foods high in, 110